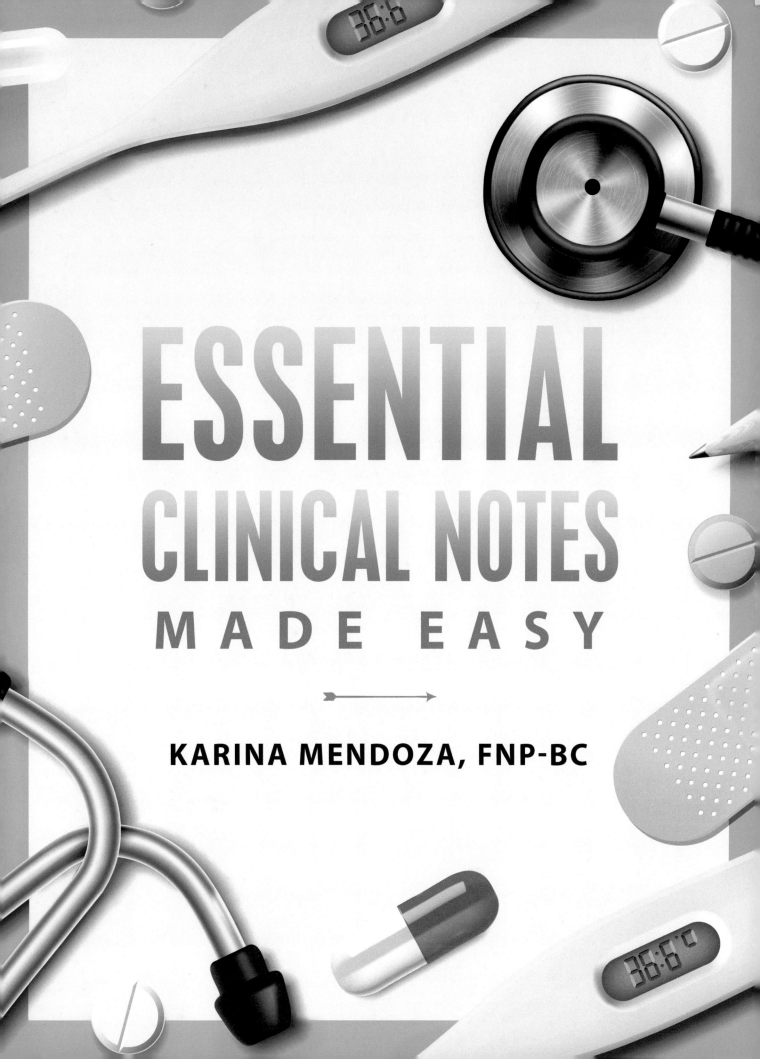

ESSENTIAL
CLINICAL NOTES
MADE EASY

→

KARINA MENDOZA, FNP-BC

Balboa Press books may be ordered through booksellers or by contacting:

Balboa Press
A Division of Hay House
1663 Liberty Drive
Bloomington, IN 47403
www.balboapress.com
1 (877) 407-4847

Because of the dynamic nature of the Internet, any web addresses or links contained in this book may have changed since publication and may no longer be valid. The views expressed in this work are solely those of the author and do not necessarily reflect the views of the publisher, and the publisher hereby disclaims any responsibility for them.

Any people depicted in stock imagery provided by Getty Images are models, and such images are being used for illustrative purposes only.
Certain stock imagery © Getty Images.

ISBN: 978-1-9822-4387-6 (sc)
ISBN: 978-1-9822-4388-3 (e)

Library of Congress Control Number: 2020903852

Print information available on the last page.

Balboa Press rev. date: 07/22/2020

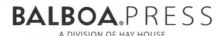

BALBOA.PRESS
A DIVISION OF HAY HOUSE

To my fellow colleagues around the world dedicating their lives for saving others. Thank you for all your efforts, devotion, strength and dedication. You are a Hero!

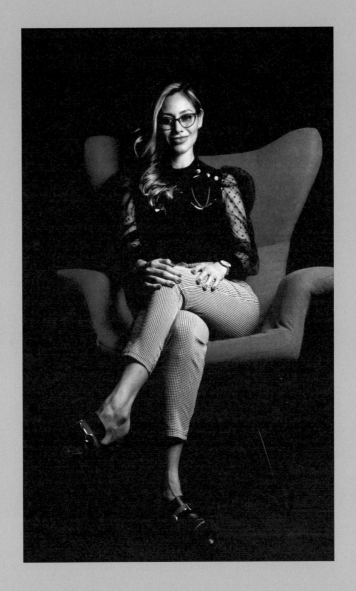

Karina Mendoza, is a Family Nurse Practitioner in El Paso,TX. She started as a Certified Nurse Assistant and decided to pursue a career in nursing after experiencing her father's death due to Cancer. As a result of this life changing event, her passion for helping others grows every day. She holds a Master's Degree in Nursing and currently pursues a Doctorate Degree in the same field. She is devoted to learn and grow to be able to help others. She is determined, grateful and passionate about life. Her life motto is "Limits exist only in the mind".

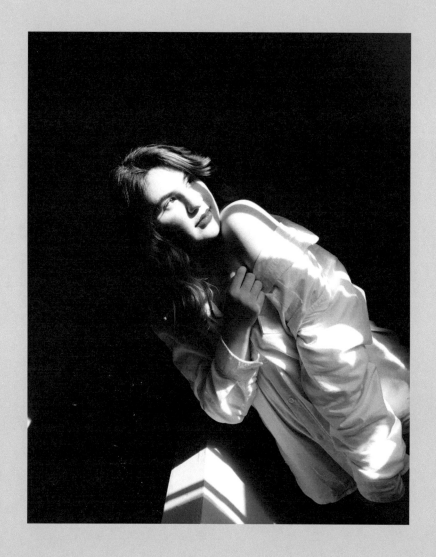

Jessica Valdivia is the artist behind Essential Clinical Notes by ClinicalExperts Choice, she is a psychology student in Mexico where she currently resides. Since she was little, she felt very connected with art thus creativity is one of her strengths when it comes to her studies. With ClinicalExperts Choice she had the great opportunity to bring together two of the things she likes most, art and health field. This book was created to invite the reader to explore another learning method to obtain knowledge, contains important information distributed in a simple way to remember the content for those who like Jessica enjoy learning in an easier and unconventional way.

index

NEUROLOGICAL DISORDERS.................

- Alzheimer
- Bell's palsy
- Cluster headaches
- Cranial nerves
- Migraine headaches
- Multiple sclerosis
- Myasthenia gravis
- Parkinson's disease
- Seizure
- Tension headaches
- Trigeminal neuralgia
- Transient ischemic attack (TIA).

ORTHOPEDIC DISORDERS........................

- Ankle sprain
- Bursitis
- Carpal tunnel syndrome
- Costochondritis
- Knee injury/pain
- Low back pain
- Muscle strain
- Morton's neuroma
- Osgood-schlatter
- Osteoarthritis
- Plantar fasciitis
- Polymyalgia rheumatica
- Rheumatoid arthitis
- Soft tissue injuries

OBSTETRIC AND PREGNANCY...........................

- Abortion
- Abrupto placentae
- Complications during pregnancy
- Contraceptive options
- Ectopic pregnancy
- Intrauterine pregnancy
- Placentia previa
- Postpartum complications
- Premature labor

PULMONARY DISORDERS....................

- Acute bronchitis
- Asthma
- COPD
- Cough etiologies and treatment
- Cystic fibrosis
- Pertussia
- Pneumonia

RESPIRATORY DISORDERS......................
- Common cold
- Influenza "flu"
- Mononucleosis
- Nose bleeds
- Pharyngitis/Tonsillitis
- Sinusitis (Rhinosinusitis)

SEXUALLY TRANSMITTED INFECTIONS/DISEASES.........
- -Acquired immune deficiency syndrome (AIDS)
- -Chancroid
- -Chlamydia
- -Genital warts (condyloma acuminata)
- -Gonorrhea
- -Hepatitis B
- -Herpes
- -Lymphogranuloma venereum LGV
- -Molluscum contagiosum
- -Syphilis

SKIN DISORDERS.......................
- Acne
- Bacterial infections
- Herpes zoster (shingles)
- Keratosis and skin cancers
- Scabies
- Other
- ***WOMEN'S HEALT***H...............
- Abnormal Uterine Bleeding
- Amenorrhea
- Breast Cancer
- Breast Cancer Screening
- Cervical Cancer Screening for Average/Risk Woman
- Dysmenorrhea
- Fibrocystic Breast Disease
- Menopause
- Pelvic Inflammatory (PID)
- Polycystic Ovarian Syndrome (PCOS)
- Premenstrual Syndrome (PMS)/ Premenstrual Dysphoric Disorder (PDD)
- Systemic Lupus Erythematosus (SLE)
- Vulvovaginitis

ANTIBIOTICS

ANTIBIOTICS
ANTIBIOTICS
ANTIBIOTICS
ANTIBIOTICS

ANTIFOLATES
CEPHALOSPORINS
FLUOROQUINOLONES
MACROLIDES
PENICILLINS
TETRACYCLINES
ANTIBIOTICS DURING
PREGNANCY

Antifolates

Common side effect: Generally well tolerated. Nausea, vomiting, skin reactions, photosensitivity; rash; pruritus.
Sulfamethoxazole/Trimethoprim (BACTRIM, SEPTRA)
Used for: UTI treatment or prophylaxis; skin and soft tissue infections; low-risk AECOPD; PJP prophylaxis.

Trimethoprim (PROLOPRIM)
Used for: UTI treatment (only 3 days needed if uncomplicated); UTI prophylaxis

Clindamycin (DALACIN C)
Used for: skin and soft tissue infections; dental infections (although usually safer options). Reduces toxin production of Streptococci and Staphylococci (e.g. useful to hypotoxic shock syndrome in necrotizing fasciitis - give in combination with penicillin).

Metronidazole (FLAGYL)
Used for: intra-abdominal infections; C. difficile; bacterial vaginosis; trichomoniasis; diabetic foot infections; fistulizing Crohn's disease (may help drainage). Chronic use may have benefit in Crohn's, but risk of AE

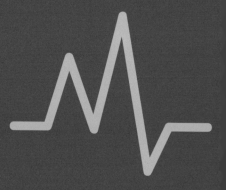

Nitrofurantoin (MACROBID)
Used for: First-line therapy in UTIs (only 5 days needed if uncomplicated). Avoid if suspected pyelonephritis.

Fosfomycin (MONUROL)
Used for: UTIs. Avoid if suspected pyelonephritis. Safe in pregnancy but usually better options.

Linezolid (ZYVOXAM)
Used for: multi-drug resistant infections (including pneumonia, skin and soft tissue, etc.).

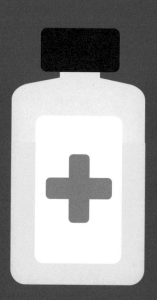

Vancomycin (VANCOCIN)
Used for: Only oral use is for treatment of Clostridium difficile colitis (drug of choice if severe infection, or if second recurrence of C. diff infection; taper over ~8wks in recurrent infections.

CEPHALOSPORINS

Common side effects: Rash, nausea, diarrhea.
Cephalexin (KEFLEX) & Cefadroxil (DURICEF)
Used for: Skin and soft tissue infections; step down option
from IV cefazolin. Take with food to reduce GI upset.

Cefprozil (CEFZIL) & Cefuroxime (CEFTIN)
Used for: low-risk AECOPD; community-acquired
pneumonia.

Cefixime (SUPRAX)
Used for: gonorrhea (800mg po x1 dose + azithro);
pyelonephritis or complicated UTIs; low-risk AECOPD.

Ceftriaxone Injection (ROCEPHIN)
Used for: One-time IM dose for gonorrhea; initial
treatment of suspected pyelonephritis while waiting for
cultures.

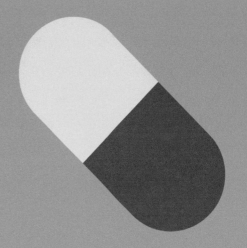

FLUOROQUINOLONES

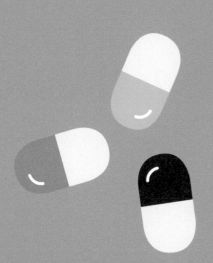

Common side effects: GI upset; rash/photosensitivity;
elevated QT; confusion/psychosis; increase or decrease
glucose; seizure; tendinopathy/tendon rupture; retinal
detachment; increase weakness in myasthenia gravis;
articular damage in kids; hepatotoxicity; nephrotoxicity.

Ciprofloxacin (CIPRO)
Used for: Pseudomonal infections; complicated UTIs;
intra-abdominal infections.

Levofloxacin (LEVAQUIN)
Used for: high-risk AECOPD; pneumonia (usually as
alternative to 1st-line agents); intra-abdominal infections.

Moxifloxacin (AVELOX)
Used for: high-risk AECOPD; pneumonia (usually as
alternative to 1st-line agents). Does not penetrate urine –
do not use to treat UTIs.

MACROLIDES

Common side effects: GI upset (erythromycin highest incidence); QT prolongation; increase LFTs; headache and insomnia.

Azithromycin (ZITHROMAX)
Used for: Pneumonia; upper respiratory tract infections; low-risk AECOPD; sexually transmitted infections including chlamydia and gonorrhea; MAC prophylaxis in HIV pts; cat-scratch disease; travelers' diarrhea (in kids, or travel to Asian countries).

Clarithromycin (BIAXIN)
Used for: Pneumonia; upper respiratory tract infections; low-risk AECOPD; MAC prophylaxis in HIV patients.

Erythromycin
upper respiratory tract infections; acne; pneumonia if sensitive pathogen is cultured; pregnancy (non-estolate formulation).

TETRACYCLINES

Common side effects: GI upset, vaginal candidiasis, photosensitivity, lightheadedness, dizziness, vertigo, ataxia, drowsiness & fatigue.

Doxycycline (DOXYCIN)
Used for: Pneumonia; low-risk AECOPD, purulent skin & soft tissue infections; ricketssia; acne; Lyme disease

Minocycline (MINOCIN)
Used for: Some prosthetic joint infections; acne.

Tetracycline (TETRACYN)
Used for: Acne; actinomycosis; periodontitis.

PENICILLINS

Common side effects: Rash, nausea, vomiting, diarrhea, melanoglossia.

Amoxicillin (AMOXIL)
Used for: Upper respiratory tract infections
Sinusitis
Acute otitis media
Dental procedure prophylaxis
Low- risk AECOPD

Amox/Clavulanate (CLAVULIN)
Used for: bite wounds; respiratory tract infections; high-risk AECOPD

Ampicillin
Used for: some UTIs with sensitive enterococcus; meningitis
Cloxacillin
Used for: Skin and soft tissue infections (MSSA). Narrow-spectrum agent; often used as step-down therapy when MSSA is known pathogen.

Penicillin V
Used for: bacterial pharyngitis; rheumatic fever prophylaxis (prophylactic dose is 250mg po q12h) q12h dosing in pharyngitis appears effective.

ANTIBIOTICS DURING PREGNANCY/ LACTATION

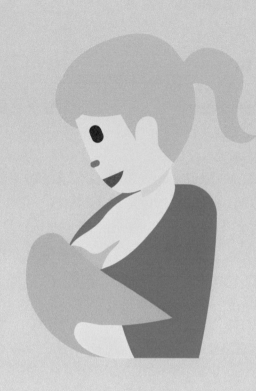

Antibiotics During Pregnancy/Lactation		Safe / Likely Safe / Caution / Contraindicated			
		1st Trimester	2nd Trimester	3rd Trimester	Lactation
FLUOROQUINOLONES		? malformations	safer alternatives usually available		
MACRO	Erythromycin – non-estolate				
	Erythromycin estolate ILOSONE	risk of maternal hepatotoxicity			
	Azithromycin / Clarithromycin				
PEN	Amoxicillin ± clav / Ampicillin	?cleft lip/palate ≤0.4%			(with clavulanate)
	Cloxacillin / Penicillin V				
CEPHALOSPORINS					
TETRACYCLINES		abnormal teeth & bone development, malformations, maternal hepatotoxicity			tetracycline doxy-, mino-cycline
OTHERS	Clindamycin				
	Cotrimoxazole SEPTRA, BACTRIM — Sulfamethoxazole			hemolytic anemia, neonate jaundice, kernicterus	ok in healthy term infants without G6PD deficiency
	Cotrimoxazole SEPTRA, BACTRIM — Trimethoprim	↓ folic acid			
	Metronidazole (oral)	1st trimester: accumulated data suggests likely safe			may hold breastfeeding 12-24hr post tx
	Nitrofurantoin			neonate hemolytic anemia	avoid in infants 8 d to 1 mons & G6PD deficiency
	Vancomycin				

PATIENT NAME:_____**DATE:**_____

Symptoms of a VIRAL INFECTION:

O *Upper respiratoyry tract infection (common cold): lasts 7-14 days*
O *Flu: lasts 7-14 days*
O *Acute pharyngitis ("sore throat"): lasts 3-7 days, upt to <10 days*
O *Acute bronchitis/Chest cold: Lasts 7-21 days*
O *Acute sinusitis: lasts 7-14 days*

You have not been prescribed antibiotcs because antibiotics are **NOT EFFECTIVE IN TREATING VIRAL INFECTIONS**, can cause side effects and may even cause serious harm.

When you have a viral infection it is very important to get plenty of rest and give your body time to fight off the virus by following these instructions:

- Rest as much as possible
- Drink plenty of fluids
- Wash your hands frequently
- Take over-the-counter medication, as advised:

O *Acetaminophen (e.g. Tylenol) for fever*
O *Ibuprofen (e.g. Advil) for fever and aches*
O *Naproxen (e.g. Aleve) for fever and aches*
O *Lozenge (cough candy) for sore throat*
O *Nasal spray (e.g. Salinex, Flonase, Nasacort or Otrivin) for nasal stuffiness*
O *Other:* _____

RETURN TO YOUR PROVIDER IF:

-Symptoms do not improve in _____ day(s), or worsen at any time
-You develop a high fever (above 38 C, or _____as directed)
-Other: _____

CARDIOVASCULAR
DISORDERS

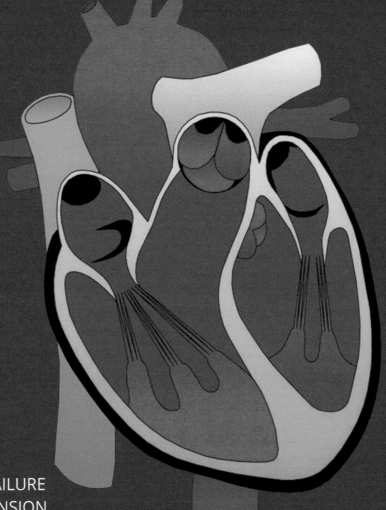

HEART FAILURE
HYPERTENSION
MURMURS
VALVULAR DISEASE : MAJOR
PROBLEMS

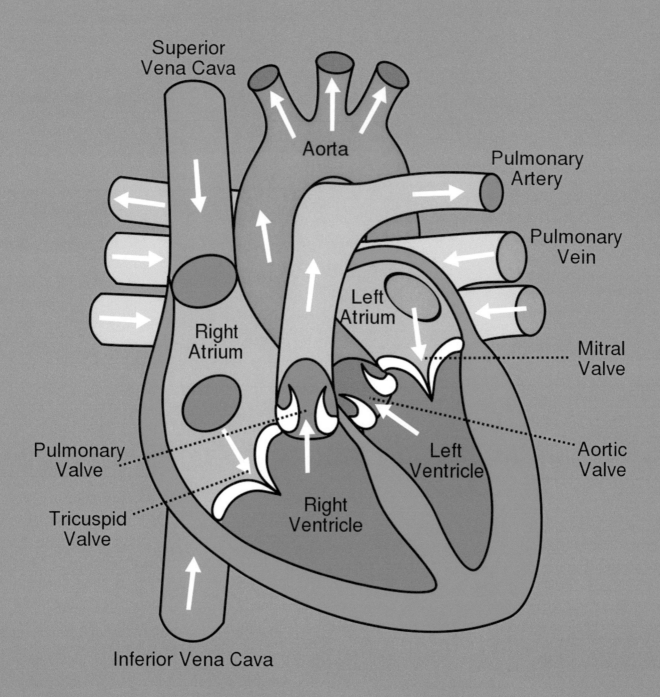

MURMURS:

I/VI: Barely audible

II/VI: Audible but faint

III/VI: Moderately loud, easily heard

IV/VI: Loud, associated with a thrill

V/IV: Very loud, heard with one corner of the stethoscope off the chest wall

VI/VI: Loudest

heart failure

A syndrome that results when the cardiac output is insufficient to meet the metabolic needs of the body

TYPES OF HEART FAILURE:

- **Systolic:** inability to contract results in decreased cardiac output
- **Diastolic:** inability to relax and fill results in decreased cardiac output
- **Acute:** abrupt onset usually follows acute MI or valve rupture
- **Chronic:** develops as a result of inadequate compensatory mechanisms that have been employed over time to improve cardiac output

SIGNS/SYMPTOMS (Acute): Left failure

1. Dyspnea at rest
2. Coarse rales over all lung fields
3. Wheezing, frothy cough
4. Appears generally healthy except for the acute event
5. S3 gallop
6. Murmur of mitral regurgitation (systolic murmur loudest at apex)

SIGNS/SYMPTOMS (Chronic): Right failure:

1. JVD
2. Hepatomegaly, splenomegaly
3. Dependent edema as a result of high capillary hydrostatic pressure
4. Paroxysmal nocturnal dyspnea (PND)
5. Appears chronically ill
6. Diffuse chest wall heave
7. Displaced PMI
8. Abdominal fullness
9. Fatigue on exertion
10. S3 and/or S4

New York Heart Association (NYHA) Functional Classification of Heart Failure

NYHA CLASS	Manifestations
I	No limitations of physical activitY
II	Slight limitations of physical activity but comfortable at rest
III	Marked limitations of physical activity but comfortable at rest
IV	Severe, inability to carry out any physical activity without discomfort

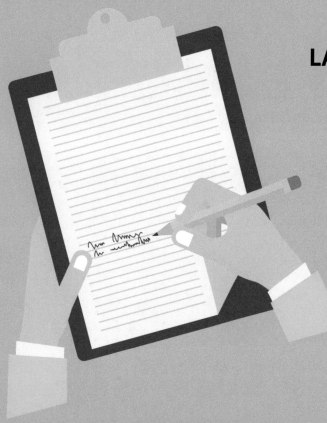

LABORATORY DIAGNOSTICS:

1. Hypoxemia and hypocapnia on ABG
2. Basic metabolic profile usually normal unless chronic failure is present
3. Urinalysis
4. Chest x-ray: pulmonary edema, Kerley B lines, effusions
5. Echocardiogram will show contractile/relaxation, valve function, ejection fraction
6. ECG may show deviation or underlying problem: acute myocardial infracion, dysrhythmia
7. Pulmonary function tests for wheezing during exercise

TREATMENT

NON- PHARMACOLOGIC
1. Sodium restriction
2. Rest/ activity balance
3. Weight reduction
4. Others

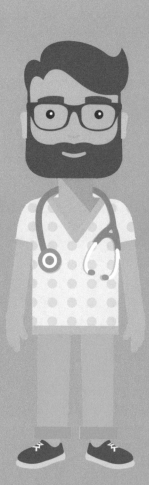

PHARMACOLOGIC:
1. ACE inhibitiors
2. Diuretics: thiazides, loop, etc
3. Anticoagulation therapy for atrial fibrillation

HYPERTENSION

Exacerbating factor: smoking, obesity, excessive alcohol intake, use of NSAIDS, and others.

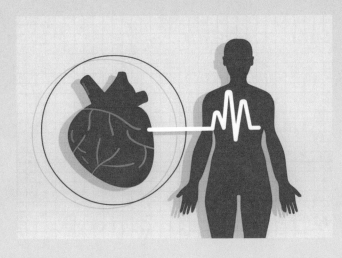

SYMPTOMS:

1. Often none: silent killer
2. Elevated BP
3. With severe hypertension: suboccipital pulsating headache, occurring early in the morning and resolving throughout the day
4. Epistaxis
5. Dizziness/lightheadedness
6. S4 related to left ventricular hypertrophy
7. Areriovenous (AV) nicking
8. Tearing chest pain may indicate aortic dissection

LABORATORY DIAGNOSTICS:

1. Uncomplicated hypertension, laboratory findings are usually normal
2. Other tests to rule out particular causes:
- Renovascular disease studies
- Chest x-ray (CXR) if cardiomegaly is suspected
- Plasma aldosterone level to rule out aldosteronism
- A.M./P.M. cortisol levels to rule out Cushing's Syndrome
3. U/A, CBC, BMP, calcium, phosphorus, uric acid, cholesterol, triglycerides
4. Electrocardiography (ECG)
5. PA and lateral CXR

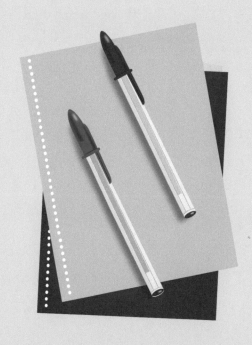

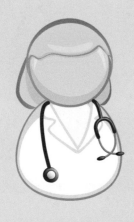

BP CATEGORY	ACC/AHA (2017-2018)	
	SBP	DBP
NORMAL	<120	<80
ELEVATED	120-129	<80
HYPERTENSION		
STAGE 1	130-139	80-89
STAGE 2	>140	>90

TREATMENT (NON-PHARMACOLOGIC):

1. Restrict sodium
2. Weight loss, if overweight
3. DASH (dietary approaches to stop hypertension)
4. Exercise (aerobic exercise 30-40 minutes each day)
5. Stress management planning
6. Reduction or elimination of alcohol
7. Smoking cessation
8. Maintenance of adequate potassium, calcium, and magnesium intake

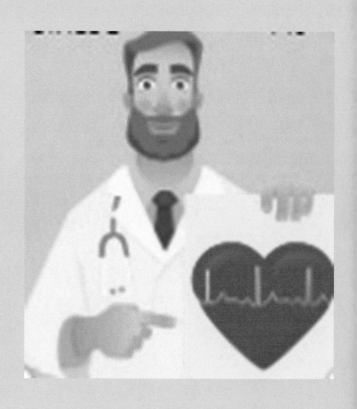

murmurs

1. *Where?*
a) 5th ICS: Apex : Mitral
b) 2nd or 3rd ICS: Base: Aortic

2. *When?*
a) Systole?
b) Diastole?

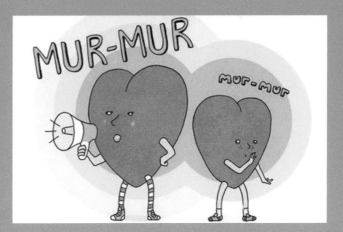

Mitral   **M**itral
Stenosis   **R**egurgitation
Aoritc   **A**ortic
Regurgtation   **S**tenosis
Diastolic   **S**ystolic

valvular disease: major problems

1. <u>**Mitral stenosis:**</u> loud S1 murmur pitched, low pitched, mid-diastolic, apical "crescendo" rumble
2. <u>**Mitral regurgitations**</u>: S3 with systolic murmur at 5th ICS MCL (apex), may radiate to base or left axilla: musical, blwing, or high pitched
3. <u>**Aortic stenosis:**</u> systolic, "blowing", rough harsh murmur at 2nd right ICS usually radiating to the neck
4. <u>**Aortic rgurgitation:**</u> diastolic, "blowing" murmur at 2nd left ICS
5. "Ms. ard and Mr. ass"

ENDOCRINE DISORDERS

Addison's disease
Cushing's disease
Diabetes Mellitus TYPE 1
Diabetes Mellitus TYPE 2
Hyperparathyroidism
Hypoparathyroidism
Hyperthyroidism
Hypothyroidsm
Hypoglycemia

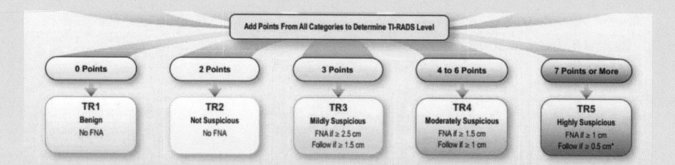

Add Points From All Categories to Determine TI-RADS Level				
0 Points	2 Points	3 Points	4 to 6 Points	7 Points or More
TR1	**TR2**	**TR3**	**TR4**	**TR5**
Benign	Not Suspicious	Mildly Suspicious	Moderately Suspicious	Highly Suspicious
No FNA	No FNA	FNA if ≥ 2.5 cm	FNA if ≥ 1.5 cm	FNA if ≥ 1 cm
		Follow if ≥ 1.5 cm	Follow if ≥ 1 cm	Follow if ≥ 0.5 cm*

ADDISON'S DISEASE

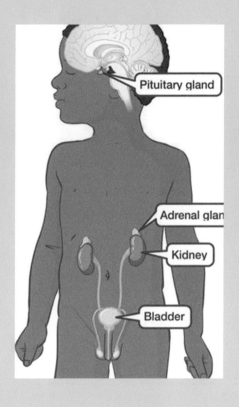

CAUSES

-Metastatic cancer
-Bilateral adrenal hemorrhage
-Pituitary failure

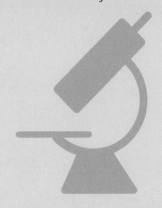

SIGNS AND SYMPTOMS

Hyperpigmentation in buccal mucosa
-Diffuse tanning and freckles
-Orthostasis and hypotension
- Scant axillary and pubic hair

LABORATORY DIAGNOSTICS

· Hypoglycemia
· Hyponatremia
· Hyperkalemia
· Elevated ESR
· Lymphocytosis
· Plasma cortisol <5 mcg/dL
· Cosyntropin

TREATMENT

-Specialist referral
-Glucocorticoid and mineralocorticoid replacement
(Hydrocortisone, Fludrocortisone acetate)

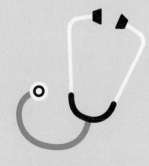

CRUSHING'S
SYNDROME

● ●

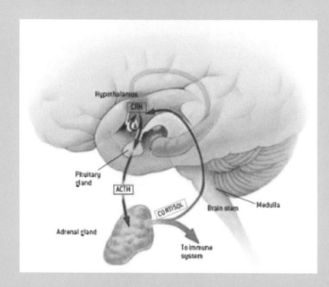

CAUSES:

ACTH hypersecretion by the pituitary
-Adrenal tumors
-Chronic administration of glucocorticoids

LABORATORY DIAGNOSTICS:

Hyperglycemia
-Hypernatremia
-Hypokalemia
-Glycosauria
-Leukocytosis
-Elevated plasma cortisol in the a.m.
-Dexamethasone suppression test to differentiate cause
-Serum ACTH

SIGNS AND SYMPTOMS:

–Central obesity
-Moon face with buffalo hump
- Acne
-Poor wound healing
-Purple striae
-Hirsutism
-Hypertension
-Weakness
-Amenorrhea
-Impotence
-Headache
-Polyuria and thirst
-Labile mood
-Frequent infections

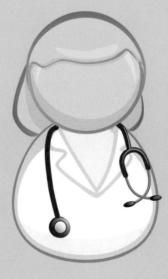

TREATMENT:

-Manage electrolyte balance
-Treat the baseline cause

DIABETES MELLITUS TYPE 1 DM

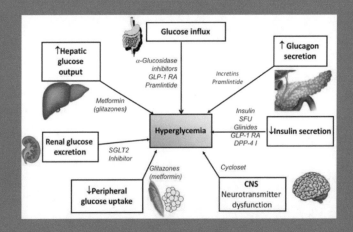

Insulin dependent or juvenile diabetes

SIGNS AND SYMPTOMS:

1. Polyuria
2. Polydipsia
3. Polyphagia
4. Nocturnal enuresis
5. Weight loss
6. Weakness/fatigue

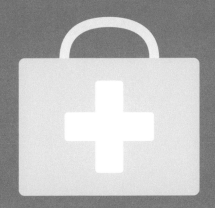

SIGNS AND SYMPTOMS:

1. Insidious inset of hyperglycemia patient may be asymptomatic
2. Polyuria
3. Polydipsia
4. Recurrent vaginitis often first symptom in women
5. Peripheral neuropathies
6. Blurred vision
7. Chronic skin infections including pruritus

DIAGNOSTIC STUDIES

· Serum fasting
· Random plasma glucose
· Glycated hemoglobin (AIC) > 6.5%

DIABETES MELLITUS TYPE 2 DM

PATHOLOGY: Inadequate to meet the patient's insulin needs

DIAGNOSTIC STUDIES

Serum fasting. Random plasma glucose. HA1C> 6.5%

TREATMENT

Weight control, dietary treatment and exercise

MONOTHERAPY FOR TYPE 2

I. Metformin

II. GLP-1 Receptor agonist

III. SGLT-2 Inhibitor

IV. DPP-4 Inhibitor

V. Alpha-Glucosidase inhibitor

VI. Thiazolidinedione (use with caution)

VII. Sulfonamide (use with caution)

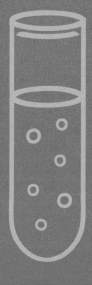

HYPERPARATHYROIDISM

Excess parathyroid hormone (PTH) secretion

SIGNS AND SYMPTOMS:

1. Asymptomatic hypercalcemia
2. Selective cortical bone loss
3. Fatigue
4. Depression
5. Bone and joint pain
6. Muscle weakness
7. Anorexia, vomiting
8. Kidney stones

DIAGNOSTIC STUDIES:

· Elevated intact plasma PTH with elevated calcium
· Hypophosphatemia

TREATMENT

-Parathyroidectomy
-Vitamin D-2
-Biophosphonates
-Hormone replacement therapy for post-menopausal women with signs of osteoporosis

HYPOPARATHYROIDISM

Insufficient parathyroid (PTH) secretion

SIGNS AND SYMPTOMS:

1. Hypocalcemia
2. Patchy hair loss
3. Fatigue
4. Anxiety or depression
5. Painful menstruation
6. Hoarseness or dyspnea
7. Paresthesias
8. Seizures

DIAGNOSTIC STUDIES:

· Decreased PTH with decreased calcium
· Hyperphosphatemia

TREATMENT

-Calcium cabonate
-High doses of vitamin D
-Once daily injection or parathyroid hormone (Natpra) for severe cases

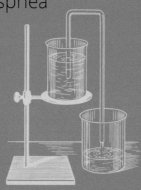

hyperthyroidism

SYMPTOMS

1. Nervousness
2. Anxiety
3. Increased sweating
4. Fatigue
5. Emotional liability
6. Fine temors
7. Increased appetite
8. Weight loss
9. Fine/thin hair
10. Lid lag
11. Tachycardia
12. Heat intolerance
13. Increased incidence of atrial fibrillation

DIAGNOSTIC STUDIES
-TSH
-T3, T4 Increased

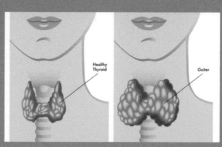

TREATMENT

-Specialist referral
-Propranolol (Inderal) for symptomatic relief:
Begin dosing with 10 mg p.o.,
may go to 80 mg four times daily

hypothyroidism

DIAGNOSTIC STUDIES
· TSH: Elevated
· T4: Low or low normal
· Resin T3 uptake: Decreased
· Hyponatremia
· Hypoglycemia

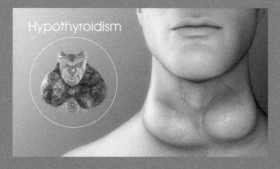

Hypothyroidism

TREATMENT

Levothyroxine

SYMPTOMS

1. Extreme weakness
2. Muscle fatigue
3. Arthralgias
4. Cramps
5. Cold intolerance
6. Constipation
7. Weight pain
8. Dry skin
9. Hair loss
10. Brittle nails
11. Puffy eyes
12. Edema of the hands and face
13. Bradycardia
14. Hypoactive bowel sounds

Hypoglycemia

SYMPTOMS

Symptoms are sudden and range from mild to severe:
- Excessive sweating
- Tiredness, lightheadedness
- Feeling dizzy and weak
- Being pale
- A sudden feeling of excess hunger
- Increased heart rate
- Blurred vision
- Confusion
- Irritable or nervous

SYMPTOMS OF HYPOGLYCEMIA DURING SLEEP INCLUDE:

- Having nightmares
- Crying in sleep
- Excessive sweating so as to dampen your clothes
- Feeling tired, irritated or confused after waking up

Severe cases can lead to:
- Convulsions/seizures
- Delirium
- Fainting
- Loss of consciousness

CAUSES

Taking higher doses of certain antidiabetic medications such as insulin, sulphopnylureas (for example, glibenclamide, gliclazide), prandial glucose regulators (for example, repaglinide, nateglinide)
Medications such as antimalarial drugs
Delayed or skipping meals
Not consuming enough carbohydrates
Over exercising
Consumption of alcohol
Medical conditions such as hepatitis, kidney problems
Diseases of pancreas such as tumors that can lead to increased production of insulin
Deficiency of certain hormones involved in glucose metabolism e.g., cortisone

PREVENTION

- Monitor blood sugar
- Keep track on medications to avoid taking double doses
- Know the signs and symptoms of hypoglycemia
- Treat underlying causes

COMPLICATIONS

Extreme (or prolonged) hypoglycemia can lead to coma and death.

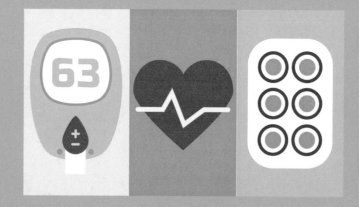

TREATMENT OF HYPOGLYCEMIA INVOLVES:

Immediate initial treatment to raise your blood sugar level
Early symptoms can usually be treated by consuming 15 to 20 grams of a fast-acting carbohydrate, such as a juice. Recheck blood sugar after 15 minutes. Repeat until patient is able to eat a full meal. If patient is unconscious or unable to drink or eat send patient to nearest emergency room.
Treatment of the underlying condition that's causing your hypoglycemia to prevent it from recurring

ENT
disorders

Acute otitis media and serous
otitis media
Otitis Externa
Blepharitis
Chalazion
Cholesteatoma
Conjunctivitis
Hearing loss
Hordeolum (STYE)
Retinal detachment
Vertigo

Acute Otitis Media & Serous Otitis Media

Presence of fluid in the middle ear accompanied by signs/symptoms of infection.

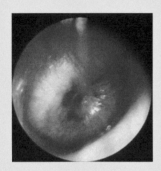

SEROUS OTITIS MEDIA
· Chronic otitis media often resulting in effusion
· The most common cause is URI (often viral)

TREATMENT:
-Uncomplicated cases resolve spontaneously or with hydration, oral decongestants, cool mist humidifiers.
-Antibiotic therapy only for suspected bacterial cases: amoxicillin-clavulanate

SIGNS AND SYMPTOMS:
1. Otalgia (slight to severe), spreading to the temporal region
2. Otorrhea
3. Vertigo
4. Nystagmus
5. Tinnitus
6. Fever
7. Lethargy
8. Nausea and omitting
9. Anorexia
10. Local inflammation: erythema with diminished light reflex, fluid in middle ear
11. Exudative phase: middle ear serous exudate
12. Suppurative phase: purulent exudates

Otitis Externa

Inflammation and/or infection of the external auditory canal (and/or auricle and tympanic membrane).

ACUTE LOCALIZED FURUNCULOSIS
CAUSE: *STAPHYLOCOCCUS AUREUS*
A. Pustules and furuncles in the outer third of the ear canal
B. Crusting
C. Severe pain (otalgia) with area of cellulitis
D. Fissuring
E. Itching
F. Possible exudates
G. Erythema
H. Scaling

TREATMENT:
Cleansing and debridement of the ear.
Topical otic drops: cortisporin otic.
Pain control: NSAID's, topical corticosteroids

BLEPHARITIS......................

Staphylococcus infection or seborrheic dermatitis of the lid edge.

SIGNS AND SYMPTOMS:
1. Red, scaly, greasy flakes
2. Thickened, crusted lid margins
3. Burning
4. Itching
5. Tearing

TREATMENT:
-Hot compresses.
-Topical antibiotics: Bacitracin or erythromycin
-Vigorously scrub lashes and lid margins with eyes closed and follow with thorough rinsing

.... CHALAZION

SIGNS AND SYMPTOMS;
-Swelling on the eye lid
-Eyelid tenderness
-Sensitivity to light
-Increased tearing
-If very large: may cause astigmatism due to pressure on the cornea

-Beady nodule on the eye lid, infection or retention cyst of a meibomian gland, usually in the upper eye lid.
-Usually painless, tenderness caused from localized swelling.

CHOLESTEATOMA ....

-Chronis otitis media consisting of peeling layers of scaly or keratinized epithelium.
-If untreated may erode the middle ear (nerve damage and deafness)

SIGN AND SYMPTOMS
Squamous epithelium lined sac, filled with desquamated keratin
Chronic infection
Painless otorrhea either unremitting or frequently recurrent
Hearing loss (ossicular damage)
Canal filled with mocopus and granulation tissue
Tympanic membrane perforation (90% of cases)

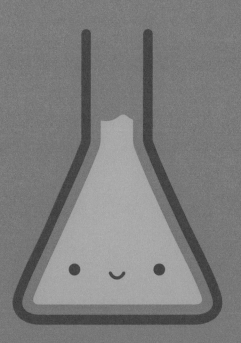

CONJUNCTIVITIS

Inflammation/ infection of the conjunctiva ("pink eye")

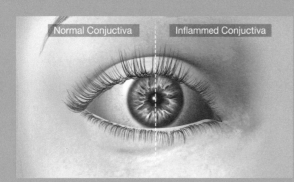

Normal Conjuctiva | Inflammed Conjuctiva

SIGNS AND SYMPTOMS:
1. Itching
2. Burning
3. Redness
4. Increased tearing
5. Blurred vision
6. Swelling of eyelids
7. Sensation of a foreign body in the eye
8. Eyelids may show a crust of sticky, mucopurulent discharge

TREATMENT:
Cortisporin ophthalmic 2gtt Q6H for 7 days

HEARING LOSS

Loss of the ability to detect pure tones in decibels > 20dB

CONDUCTIVE CAUSES	
Foreign body in the ear	Hematoma
Otitis externa	Perforated tympanic membrane
Otitis media	Otosclerosis
SENSORINEURAL CAUSES	
Damage to hair cells and/or nerves that sense sound waves	Acoustic trauma
Barotrauma (usually in divers)	Head trauma
Ototoxic drugs: Aminoglycosides, diuretics, salicylates, NSAIDS, antineoplastic	Meniere's disease
Acoustic neuroma	Infections: Mumps, measles, herpes zoster, syphilis, meningitis, etc.

LABORATORY STUDIES:
1. Otoscopic exam: inspect canal and tympanic membrane
2. General neurological exam
3. Audiometry testing
4. CT scan, if neurologic condition is suspected
5. Serum blood tests as needs

TREATMENT:
·Conductive hearing loss:
a) clear canal
b) treat underlying cause
·Sensorineural hearing loss: refer

hordeolum (stye)

Acute inflammatory, most commonly infectious, process affecting the eyelid. Usually caused by Staphylococcus aureus

SIGNS AND SYMPTOMS:
1. Abrupt pain and erythema of the eyelid.
2. Localized , tender mass developing in the eyelid

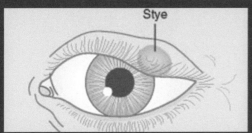

TREATMENT:
-Hot compresses
-Oral antibiotics for preseptal cellulitis (clindamycin or TMP-SMX plus amoxicillin-clavulanic acid or cefpodoxime or cefdinir)
-Refer to ophthalmologist if not resolved in 2 days

vertigo

COMMON CAUSES
Brain tumors
Medications
Otitis media or labyrinthitis
Meniere's disease
Acoustic neuroma
Head trauma or neck injury
Migraines
Cerebellar hemonthage

SIGNS AND SYMPTOMS
Sensation of disorientation or motion
Nausea or vomiting
Abnormal eye movement (nystagmus)
Hearing loss
Tinnitus
Visual disturbances
Weakness, difficulty walking
Difficulty speaking
Decreased of level of consciousness

LABORATORY DIAGNOSTICS
CT scan
VDRL/RPR
Serum medication levels
Hearing examination
Blood glucose and ECG may be helpful

TREATMENT
Diazepam (Valium)
Meclizine hydrochloride (Antivert)
Diphenhydramine (Benadryl)
Scopolamine transdermal patch
Antiemetics

retinal detachment

SIGNS AND SYMPTOMS:
1. Flashes of light (photopsia), especially in peripheral vision.
2. Floaters in the eye
3. Blurred vision
4. Shadow or blindness in a part of the visual field of one eye

TREATMENT: Referral to surgery

gastrointestinal
DISORDERS

Appendicitis
Bowel Obstruction
Cholecystitis
Colon cancer
Diverticulitis
Gastroenteritis
Gastroesophageal reflux (GERD)
Hepatitis
Irritable bowel syndrome
Peptic Ulcer disease
Ulcerative colitis

APPENDICITS

Inflammation of the appendix, if untreated, gangrene and perforation may develop within 36 hours

SYMPTOMS:
Vague, colicky umbilical pain
Pain right lower quadrant
Nausea with 1 to 2 episodes of vomiting
Pain worsened and localized with coughing

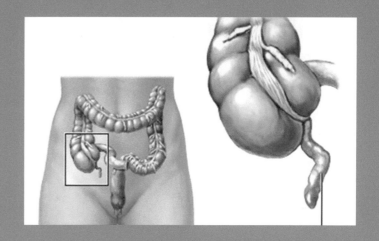

PHYSICAL FINDINGS:
1. **Right lower quadrant guarding with rebound tenderness**
2. **Psoa's signs (pain with right thigh extension)**
3. **Obstrurator sign (pain with internal rotation of flexed right thigh**
4. **Positive Rovsing's sign (right lower quadrant pain when pressure is applied to the left lower quadrant**
5. **Low grade fever**

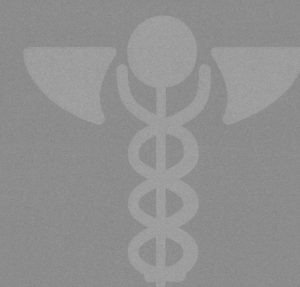

LABORATORY DIAGNOSTICS:
WBC's 10,000-20,000/mL
CT or ultrasound is diagnostic

TREATMENT:
Refer for surgical treatment and pain management

BOWEL OBSTRUCTION

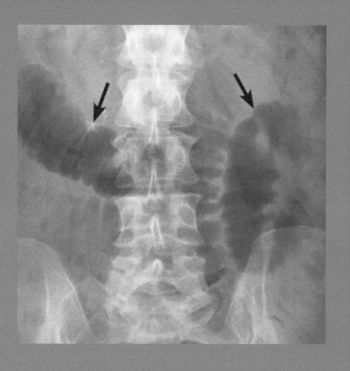

Blockage of the intestinal impeding passage of bowed contents

CAUSES:
Hernia
Adhesions
Volvulus
Tumors
Fecal impaction
Heus (functional obstruction)

PHYSICAL FINDINGS:
Abdominal distention
High pitched, tinkling bowel sounds
Unable to pass stool/gas

SYMPTOMS:
Cramping periumbilical pain initially: later becomes constant and diffuse
Vomitng

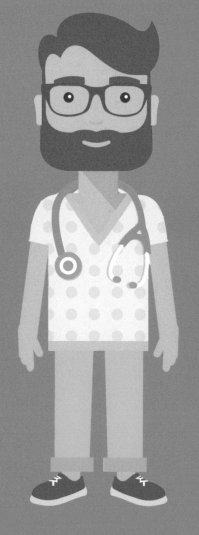

LABORATORY DIAGNOSTICS:
May see elevated WBC's and values consistent with dehydration

CHOLECYSTITIS

Inflammation of the gallbladder, associated with gallstones in >90% of cases

SYMPTOMS
1. Often precipitated by a large or fatty meal
2. Severe pain in epigastrium or right hypochondrium
3. Vomiting in many clients affords relief

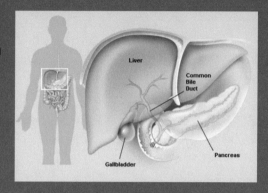

PHYSICAL FINDINGS:
A. Murphy's sign
B. Right upper quadrant tenderness to palpitation
C. Muscle guarding and rebound pain
D. Fever

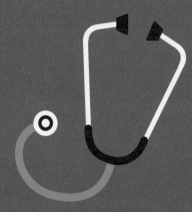

LABORATORY/DIAGNOSTICS:
WBC's serum bilubrin, AST, ALT, LDH and amylase may be elevated
Ultrasound: gold standard

TREATMENT
Pain management
For acutely ill patients, refer for GI/ surgical consult

COLON CANCER

SYMPTOMS:
-Often asymptomatic
-Changes in bowel habit
-Thin stools
-Weight loss

DIAGNOSTICS:
Stool may be guaiac positive
Colonoscopy
CBC
Carcinoembryonic antigen
(CEA) elevated

TREATMENT:
Surgical consult,
oncology consult
Supportive care

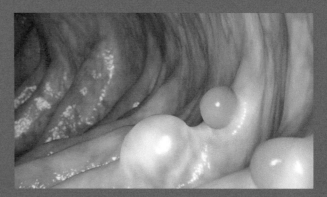

DIVERTICULITIS

Inflammation or localized perforation of diverticula with
abscess formation

SYMPTOMS:
-Mild to moderate aching abdominal pain in
left lower quadrants
-Constipation or loose stools may be present
Nausea and vomiting

PHYSICAL FINDINGS:
Low grade fever
Left lower quadrant tenderness to
palpitation
Patients with perforation present with a
more dramatic picture and peritoneal
signs

DIAGNOSTICS:
Mild to moderate leukocytosis
Elevated ESR
CT scan to evaluate abscess

TREATMENT:
NPO dependent upon condition
Refer to ER

GASTROENTERITIS

Acute nausea, vomiting, diarrhea, and cramping resulting from an acute inflammation/irritation of the gastric mucosa

SYMPTOMS:
Nausea/vomiting
Watery diarrhea
Anorexia
Abdominal cramping
General "sick" feeling

PHYSICAL EXAM FINDINGS:
Abdominal distention
Fever
Tachycardia
Hypotension
Hyperactive bowel

TREATMENT:
Fluids for rehydration
Antibiotics if symptoms are not resolved

GASTROESOPHAGEAL REFLUX (GERD)

SYMPTOMS:
"Burning;;
Hiccough
Excessive salivation
Occurs at night and/or in recumbent position
May be relieved by sitting up, antiacids, water or food

TREATMENT:
Elevate head of bed
Avoid alcohol, caffeine, spices, peppermint
Antiacids PRN
H2 blockers
Proton pump inhibitors

DIAGNOSTICS:
Consider referral for esophagogastroduodenoscopy (EGD): rule out cancer, Barret's esophagus, peptic ulcer disease, etc.

HEPATITIS

Inflammation of the liver with resultant liver dysfunction

hepatitis A

Enteral virus, transmitted via the oral-fecal route and, rarely, parenterally

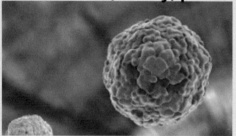

hepatitis B

Blood DNA virus present in serum, saliva, semen and vaginal secretions

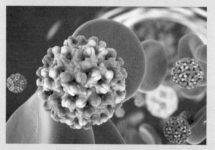

hepatitis C

Blood borne RNA virus in which the source of infection is often uncertain

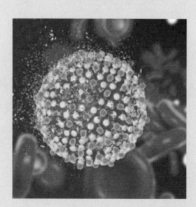

symptoms:

Pre-icteric: fatigue, malaise, anorexia, headache
Icteric: weight loss, jaundice, pruritus right upper quadrant pain, clay colored stool, dark urine
Low-grade fever may be present
Hepatosplenomegaly may be present

diagnostics:

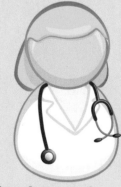

WBC low to normal
UA: proteinuria, bilirubrinuria
Elevated AST and ALT
LDH, alkaline photosphatase and PT normal or slightly elevated

Irritable Bowel Syndrome

CAUSES:
Stress theory
Greater incidence among women

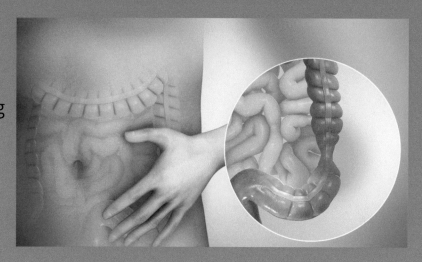

SYMPTOMS:
Abdominal cramping
Abdominal pain may be relieved by defecation
Changes in stool consistency and/or pattern
Dyspepsia
Fatigue
Complaints of anxiety and/or depression are common

DIAGNOSTICS:
Sigmoidoscopy
Barium studies

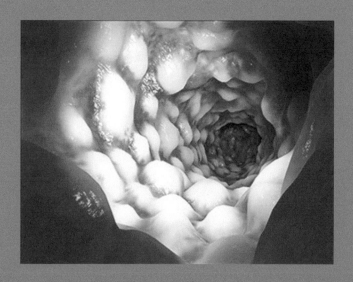

TREATMENT:
Refer to counseling and therapy as needes
High fiber diet
SSRI's for patients who are depressed
Anticholinergics, antidiarrheals, and/or antidepressant agents as warranted

PEPTIC ULCER

CAUSES:
H.pylori
NSAID's, ASA, and glucocorticoids
More common in men
More common in smokers

SYMPTOMS:
Gnawing epigastric pain
Relief of pain with eating (duodenal)
Pain worsens with eating (gastric)

LABORATORY DIAGNOSTICS
1. Normal: may note anemia on th CBC
2. Consider endoscopy after 8 to 12 weeks of treatment
3. Consider H. pylori testing

MUCOSAL PROTECTIVE AGENTS
Give 2 hours apart from other medications
1. Bismuth subsalicylate (pepto-bismol)
2. Misoprostol (cytotec) 4 times daily with food

Out-Patient Management
H2 Recetor Antagonists
Proton Pump Inhibitors 30 minutes before meals

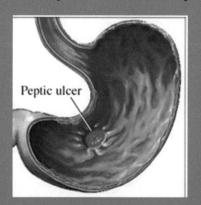
Peptic ulcer

H. PYLORI ERADICATION THERAPY:
2 antibiotics + either a proton pump inhibitor or bismuth
Metronidazole (Flagyl) 500 mg twice a day with meals, omeprazole (prilosec) 20 mg BID before meals, and amoxicillin 1 g twice a day with meals for 7 to 14 days

ULCERATIVE COLITIS

Idiopathic inflammatory characterized by diffuse mucosal inflammation of the colon

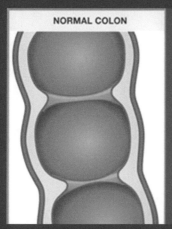
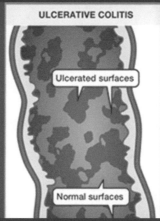

SYMPTOMS:
Bloody diarrhea is the hallmark symptom
Rectal tenesmus

DIAGNOSTIC STUDIES:
Stool studies are negative
Sigmoidoscopy

TREATMENT:
Mesalamine (Canasa) suppositories or enemas for 3 to 12 weeks
Hydrocortisone suppositories and enemas

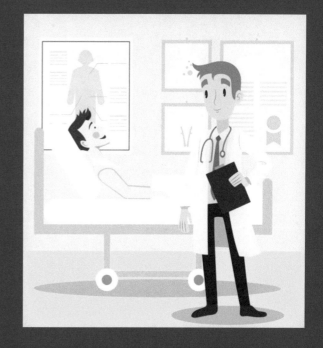

GENITOURINARY TRACT DYSFUNCTION

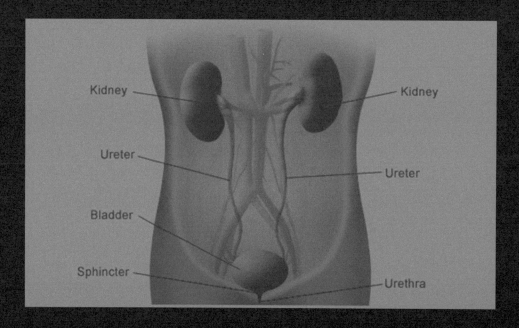

Kidney — Kidney

Ureter — Ureter

Bladder

Sphincter — Urethra

Acute Pyelonephritis
Urinary incontinence
Urinary tract infections (UTI's)

Acute Pyelonephritis

SYMPTOMS

1. Flank, low back, or abdominal pain may be present
2. Fever and chills often present and usually indicate upper UTI
3. Nausea/vomiting
4. Mental status changes in the elderly

LABORATORY/DIAGNOSTICS

1. White blood cell casts seen on urinalysis
2. ESR elevated with pyelonephritis

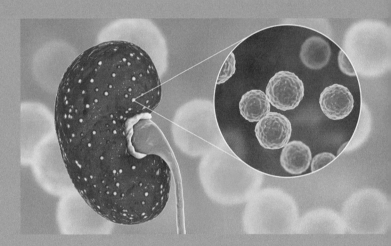

TREATMENT

1. IDSA guidelines for empiric treatment of pyelonehritis
2. a) Recommended: Ciprofloxacin 500 mg every hour hours (7 days if uncomplicated)
3. b) Levofloxacin - OK, but not Moxifloxacin
4. c) Ceftriaxone 1 mg IV every 24 hours (14 days)
5. 2. Not recommended: TMP-SMX (high resistance) or nitrofurantoin (does not get penetrate kidney)

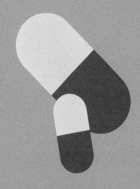

URINARY INCONTINENCE

TYPES

1. **STRESS (URETHRAL INCOMPETENCE)**
2. -CAUSES:
3. -Muscles impairing urethral support (most common)
4. -Intrinsic sphincter deficiencies due to pelvic surgery
5. -FINDINGS:
6. -Urine leakage from activities with increased pressure on bladder (lifting, coughing, exercise, sneezing, laughing, climbing stairs, etc)
7. **2. URGE (DETRUSOR OVERACTIVITY)**
8. -CAUSES
9. -Detrusor hyperactivity by CNS abnormalities such as strokes
10. -Infections of the GU tract
11. -Urinary stones
12. -Neoplasms
13. -Fecal impaction
14. -FINDINGS:
15. -Urgency, involuntary urinary loss, nocturia, frequency
16. -Often referred to as an "overactive bladder"

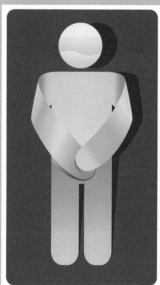
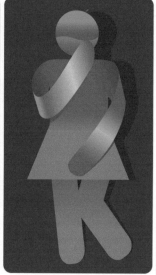

CONSIDERATIONS

Urinary incontinence is common
Associated with chronic risks such as falls and fractures

TREATMENT

1. **STRESS INCONTINENCE:**
2. -Timed voids to prevent full bladder
3. -Pessary
4. -Surgery
5. **2. URGE INCONTINENCE**
6. - Urge suppression/distraction
7. -Quick pelvic contractions
8. -Medications
9. **3. PATIENT TEACHING:**
10. -Weight loss
11. -Fluid management
12. -Avoid caffeine
13. -Bladder control: strategies
14. **4. PHARMACOTHERAPY:**
15. - Muscarinic receptor antagonists
16. *IMMEDIATE RELEASE*: Oxybutynin (Ditropan), Tolterodine (Detrol), Trospium (Sanctura)
17. *EXTENDED RELEASE*: Darifenacin (Enablex), Fesoterodine (Toviaz), Ditropan XL, Solifenacin (Vesicare), Detrol LA

URINARY TRACT INFECTIONS (UTI's)

Inflammation and infection involving the kidneys, ureters, bladder, and/or urethra

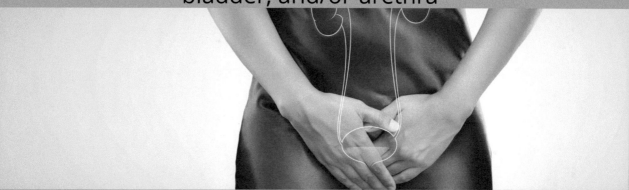

SYMPTOMS

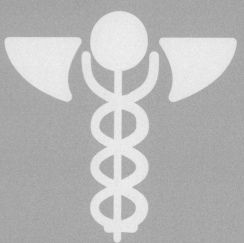

1. Dysuria is the key symptom
2. Frequency
3. Nocturia
4. Urgency
5. Hematuria- occurs in 40 to 60% of patients

LABORATORY DIAGNOSTICS

1. Urinalysis-usually shows pyuria (> 10 white blood cells/ml)
2. Presence of nitrate by dipstick is very specific but not a sensitive test for bacteriuria
3. Esterase detection by dipstick is very sensitive but not specific

TREATMENT

1. IDSA guidelines for uncomplicated cystitis (goal: low resistance and low collateral damage):
2. - Nitrofurantoin 100 mg PO BID x 5 days
3. -TMP-SMX DS PO BID x 3 days (avoid if resistance is >20%)
4. -Fosfomycin 3 gm PO x 1
5. 2. Because of the risk of serious side effects, the FDA has determined that fluoroquinolones should be reserved for use in patients who have no alternative treatment options

GROWTH &
development

Reflexes Present at Birth
- Moro
- Stepping
- Palmar
- Plantar
- Rooting
- Sucking
- Galant
- Tonic neck
- Blink, cough, gag, sneeze, yawn

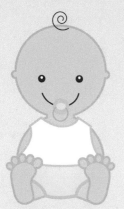

Caput succedaneum
Edema over the presenting part of the head. Resolves in a
few days. Completely benign.
Cephalohematoma (CH)
A collection of blood between a baby's scalp and the skull.
Will take weeks to resolve.
Head Circumference
- Should be plotted on a growth chart and compared to gestational age through age 3 years
- Head circumference is measured at the largest circumference, above the ears

Hearing Loss
- 0.1-0.3% of newborns have significant bilateral hearing loss
- 2-4% in the NICU
- AAP recommends universal hearing screening by age 1 month
- Goal is to detect hearing loss before 3 months of age
- Interventions by age 6 months

Babinski Reflex
- Reflex: Babinski (plantar)
- Eliciting the reflex: On sole of foot, beginning at heel, stroke upward along lateral aspect of sole, then move finger across ball of foot
- Characteristic response: All toes hyperextend, with dorsiflexion of big toe— recorded as a positive sign
- Comments: Absence requires neurological evaluation; should disappear after 1 year of age. Response depends on infant's general muscle tone, maturity, and condition

Visual Behavior
- Red reflex should be present bilaterally at birth
- If red reflex absent, consider congenital cataracts, retinoblastoma
- Vision is about 20/200 to 20/400

Ocular Discharge
- Newborn with purulent ocular discharge: Consider gonococcus, chlamydia or herpes
- Chemical conjunctivitis from erythromycin ointment 0.5% used to prevent ophthalmia neonatorum (ON) caused by gonorrhea

Ears
- Low-set ears may indicate renal agenesis
- Chromosomal abnormalities
- Assess gross hearing by observing for startle response

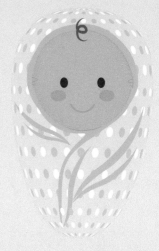

Ears
- Gross hearing of infant is assessed by observing startle response to loud noise
- Auditory brainstem response (ABR)
- Hearing loss is associated with speech and language delays

4 Months Old

Gross/Fine Motor
- Head up to 90 degrees
- No head lag when pulled upright
- Sits with head control
- Follows with eyes past midline
- Grasps rattle
- Opens hands to grasp objects
- Places hands together

Personal Social
- Smiles spontaneously
- Regards own hand

Language
- Vocalizes OOOs and AHHs
- Laughs

Fontanels
- Anterior open
- Posterior usually closed

Visual Behavior
- Intense eye contact
- Vertical and circular tracking
- Interested in mobiles
- Grasps toward hanging objects
- Disconjugate gaze

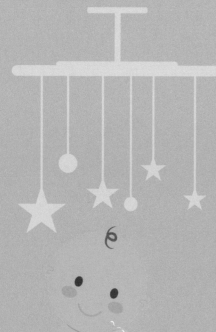

6 Months Old

Gross motor
- Length increases 0.5 inches/month
- Weight increases 3-4 oz/week
- Head circumference increases 0.25 inches/month

First Teeth
- Introduction of solid foods 2-3 times daily
- Introduce a cup

Gross/Fine Motor
- Bears weight on legs
- Lifts chest using arm support
- Rolls over
- Sits with support/maybe unsupported

Personal Social
- Works for toy
- Smiles often and interacts with caregiver

Language
- Squeals
- Turns toward rattling sound

Reflexes
- Parachute reflex appears (Infant extends arms, hands, and fingers when suspended prone and lowered quickly toward table)
- Never disappears
- Many reflexes have disappeared: Moro, stepping, rooting, palmar grasp, galant, tonic neck

Fontanels
- Anterior open

Visual Behavior
- Conjugate gaze
- Watches own hands
- Reaches toward and grasps hanging objects
- Color vision develops by 5 months

Vision Screening: Children <5 years
- Screen for strabismus:
- Strabismus is the leading cause of amblyopia
- Amblyopia: loss of vision
- When the two eyes don't focus on the same object, the brain ignores information from one of the eyes. If this is not corrected, it can result in loss of vision, amblyopia.
- The most common cause of vision problems in children
- 1%-3% have strabismus (develops between infancy and 5-7 years)

Vision Screening
- Cover-uncover test to assess for strabismus (start at age 6 months through 3 years)

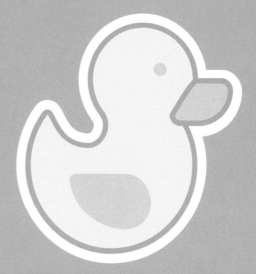

9 Months Old

Growth
- Growth is about as rapid as at 6 months
- Length increases: 0.5 inches/month
- Weight increases: 3-4 oz/week
- Head circumference increases: 0.25 inches/month

Gross/Fine Motor
- Pulls to sit
- No head lag
- Sits without support
- Crawls
- Holds to stand
- Looks for yarn
- Rakes raisin using fingers
- Passes a cube
- Creeps, crawls, and scoots
- Pulls to stand
- Bangs, shakes, throws objects
- Feeds self with fingers

Childproof Home!

Personal Social
- Feeds self with hand
- Stranger anxiety develops

Language
- Turns toward voice
- Uses single syllables
- Imitates speech sounds

Fontanels
- Anterior open but normal if closed

Visual Behavior
- Interested in pictures
- Recognizes partially hidden object

12 Months Old

Infant
- Pulls to stand, may take a few steps, "cruises"
- Bangs blocks together
- Says 2-4 words
- Feeds self and drinks from cup easily

Growth
- Length increases: 3 inches/year
- Weight increases: 4.5-6.5 pounds annually
- Weight should have tripled by this time
- Head circumference increases 1 inch annually

Gross/Fine Motor
- Pulls to stand
- Stands in 2 seconds
- Takes 2 cubes
- Thumb-finger grasp (pincer)
- Bangs 2 cubes

Personal Social
- Plays pat-a-cake

Language
- Dada, mama
- Combines syllables

Fontanels
- Anterior open but normal if closed

Visual Behavior
- Looks through window
- Recognizes people
- Recognizes pictures

15 Months Old

Gross Motor
- Stands alone
- Stoops and recovers
- Walks well

Fine Motor
- Puts block in cup

Psychosocial/ Emotional
- Indicates wants
- Waves bye bye

Language
- Jabbers
- Dada/mama specific
- Says 1 word

15-24 Months Old

Toddler
Gross/Fine Motor Skills
- Psychosocial Emotional (no longer assess Personal Social)
- Language
- Reflexes (plantar disappears 12-24 months)
- Fontanels (anterior open but OK if closed)
- Visual Acuity (conjugate gaze)

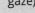
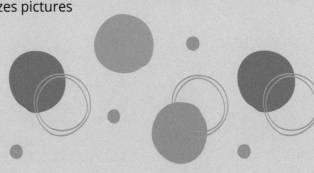

18 Months Old

Gross Motor
- ☐ Walks backward

Fine Motor
- ☐ Scribbles
- ☐ Builds tower of 2 cubes

Psychosocial/Emotional
- ☐ Plays ball with examiner
- ☐ Imitates activities
- ☐ Drinks from cup

Language
- ☐ Says 2-3 words

3 Years Old

Gross Motor
- ☐ Jumps up
- ☐ Throws ball overhand
- ☐ Rides a tricycle

Fine Motor
- ☐ Tower of 6 cubes
- ☐ Uses scissors
- ☐ Copies circle

Psychosocial/Emotional
- ☐ Puts on clothing with help
- ☐ Brushes teeth with help

Language
- ☐ Combines words
- ☐ Identifies one's picture
- ☐ Names six body parts
- ☐ Points to four pictures
- ☐ Speech half understandable

Visual Acuity
- ☐ Vision 20/50

24 Months Old

Gross Motor
- ☐ Runs
- ☐ Walks up steps
- ☐ Kicks ball forward

Fine Motor
- ☐ Dumps raisin, demonstrated
- ☐ Builds tower of 4 cubes

Psychosocial/ Emotional
- ☐ Uses spoon/fork
- ☐ Removes garments
- ☐ Feed doll

Language
- ☐ Says 6 words
- ☐ Points to picture

4 Years Old

Gross Motor
- ☐ Jumps a short distance
- ☐ Balances 2 seconds on each foot
- ☐ Catches a bouncing ball
- ☐ Throws ball underhand
- ☐ Walks down steps alternately

Fine Motor
- ☐ Copies vertical line
- ☐ Tower of 8 cubes
- ☐ Wriggles thumbs
- ☐ Dresses/undresses

Psychosocial/Emotional
- ☐ Washes/dries hands
- ☐ Names friend
- ☐ Puts on t-shirt

Language
- ☐ Knows two actions, two adjectives
- ☐ Names one color
- ☐ Uses two objects
- ☐ Counts one block
- ☐ Names four pictures

Visual Acuity
- ☐ Vision 20/40

3-5 Years Old

Preschooler
- ☐Gross/Fine Motor Skills
- ☐Psychosocial/ Emotional
- ☐ Language
- ☐ Visual Acuity (conjugate gaze)

5 Years Old

Gross Motor
- ☐ Hops
- ☐ Balances 3 seconds on each foot
- ☐ Skips
- ☐ Walks backward toe to heel
- ☐ Can somersault

Fine Motor
- ☐ Draws person in three parts
- ☐ Copies +, triangle, square
- ☐ Prints own name

Psychosocial/Emotional
- ☐ Dresses self
- ☐ Plays board games
- ☐ Brushes teeth without help
- ☐ Imaginary friend
- ☐ Shows affection
- ☐ Group play

Language
- ☐ Knows four actions
- ☐ Uses three objects
- ☐ ALL speech understandable
- ☐ Understands four prepositions
- ☐ Names four colors
- ☐ 1500-word vocabulary

Visual Acuity
- ☐ Vision 20/30

6-10 Years Old

School Age
- ☐ Gross/Fine Motor Skills
- ☐ Psychosocial Emotional
- ☐ Language
- ☐ Cognitive
- ☐ Moral Development
- ☐ Physical Development

6 Years Old

Gross Motor
- ☐ Balances
on each foot 6 seconds
- ☐ Heel-to-toe walking
- ☐ Precise and deliberate movements

Fine Motor
- ☐ Picks longer line from choices
- ☐ Copies square
- ☐ Draws person in six parts

Psychosocial/Emotional
- ☐ Prepares cereal
- ☐ Enthusiastic about surroundings
- ☐ Identifies left and right
- ☐ Some understanding of death and dying
- ☐ Wants to please

Language
- ☐ Defines five to seven words
- ☐ Knows three adjectives
- ☐ Counts five blocks
- ☐ Knows two opposites

Cognitive
- ☐ Easily disappointed and frustrated
- ☐ Reads well
- ☐ Vocabulary: 10-14K words
- ☐ Uses appropriate verb tense, word and sentence structure

Moral Development
- ☐ Understands "bad"
- ☐ Values based on others' enforced values
- ☐ Increasingly fearful of unknown

Physical Development
- ☐ Visual acuity: 20/20
- ☐ Tonsils and adenoids reach largest size
- ☐ Retina fully developed
- ☐ Eustachian tube becomes longer and more slanted
- ☐ Completely toilet trained
- ☐ Gains strength and coordination

8 Years Old

Gross Motor
- ☐ Increased physical strength and endurance

Fine Motor
- ☐ Well-developed hand-eye coordination
- ☐ Good finger control

Psychosocial/ Emotional
- ☐ Develops close circle of same-sex friends
- ☐ Enjoys group activities
- ☐ Peer pressure
- ☐ Mood swings
- ☐ Impatient

Language
- ☐ Almost able to converse at adult level
- ☐ Enjoys reading
- ☐ Understands how opposites work

Cognitive
- ☐ Desires to understand how and why things work
- ☐ Clear, logical thinking skills
- ☐ Exhibits preference for certain subjects and activities

Moral Development
- ☐ Understands "bad"
- ☐ Values based on others' enforced values
- ☐ Increasingly fearful of unknown

Physical Development
- ☐ Alveolar development complete
- ☐ Rapid maturation of endocrine system
- ☐ Long bones grow

10 Years Old

Gross Motor
- ☐ Capable of demanding motor and endurance tasks (bicycling)

Fine Motor
- ☐ Handles tools well
- ☐ Manual dexterity developed
- ☐ Capable of drawing in detail

Psychosocial/Emotional
- ☐ Dislike of opposite sex
- ☐ Generally dependable
- ☐ Same-sex friends

Language
- ☐ Continues to improve reading, comprehension, writing skills

Cognitive
- ☐ Good at memorizing, recalling info but not understanding it
- ☐ Eager to learn new skills
- ☐ Capable of concentrating and resuming task after interruption

Moral Development
- ☐ Understands right from wrong

Physical Development
- ☐ Continues with physical growth, girls may begin breast development

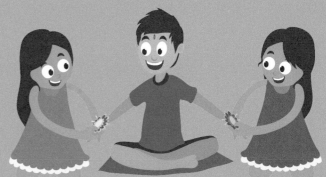

11-21 Years Old

Adolescence
 Psychosocial Emotional Development
 Cognitive
 Moral
Development
 Physical Development (Male and Female)

Early Adolescence 11-14 Years

Psychosocial/Emotional
 Concern over body image, looks, clothes
 Conflicts between high expectations and lack of confidence
 Eating problems may develop
 Peers are source for standards and models
 Interest in opposite sex
 Strives to be accepted
 Preoccupied with self
 Erratic and inconsistent behavior
Cognitive
 Strong desire to learn useful things
 Able to use logic and debate others
 Usually focuses on the present
 Prefers active learning over passive learning
 Independent critical thinking develops from arguing
Moral Development
 Tests rules and limits
 Begins to understand potential consequences of future behaviors
 Develops ideals
 Selects role models
 Experimentation: drugs, sex, alcohol, and tobacco
Male
Physical Development
 Rapid height gains (10 cm/yr)
 Ravenous appetite
 Metabolism fluctuations
 Extreme restlessness
 Body proportions similar to adult
Female
Physical Development Increased coordination and strength
 Rapid vertical growth
 Body proportions similar to adult

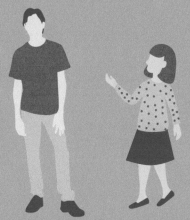

15-17 Years Old

Psychosocial/Emotional
 More interest in opposite sex
 Sex drive emerges
 Increased independence from parents
 Prefers spending time with friends
 Prone to feeling sad or depressed
 Concerned with attractiveness
 Conflicts over parental controls and independence
 Struggle for acceptance of greater authority
 Questions about sexual orientation
Cognitive
 Deeper
capacity for caring and sharing
 Develops
more intimate relationships
 Intellectual sophistication and creativity
 Increased concern with peace, poverty, and environment.
Moral Development
Questions social mores
 Understands concepts of good and evil
Male
Physical Development
 Nearing completion of vertical growth
 Acne and body odor prevalent
 Periods of excessive physical activity followed by periods of lethargy
Female
Physical Development
 Nearing completion of vertical growth
 Height completion ceases 2-2.5 years after menarche
 Acne and body odor prevalent
 Periods of excessive physical activity followed by periods of lethargy

18-21 Years Old

Late Adolescence 18-21 years
Psychosocial/Emotional
 Sets goals and follows through
 Involved in community issues
 Greater emotional stability
 Acceptance of social institutions and cultural traditions
 Greater concern for others
Cognitive
 Articulates thoughts
 Expresses ideas
 Higher level of concern for future
 Concerned about role in life
 Ability to make independent decisions
 Defined work habits
 Pride in work
 More developed sense of humor
 Ability to compromise
Moral Development
 Able to delay gratification
 Self-reliant
 Personal dignity
 Self-regulation of self-esteem
 Continued interest in moral reasoning
Male
Physical Development
 Continues to gain weight, muscle mass, and body hair
Female
Physical Development
 Fully developed

HEALTH
HEALTH
PREVENTION
PREVENTION

ADOLESCENTS
YOUNG ADULTS
MIDDLE-AGED ADULTS
ELDERLY ADULTS
OSTEOPOROSIS

adolescents

	When to start?	How often?
ADOLESCENTS (ages 11-19)		
1. Complete PE including:	11-14 years	3 visits (11-14, 15-17 and 18-21 years)
a) Height/weight (check for eating disorders)		
b) Skin exam		
c) Oral cavity		
d) Hearing		
e) Abuse/neglect/depression		
f) BP (normal = <120/80)		
2. Females:		
a) HPV	Age 9-14	Series of 2, 6 months apart or series of three at 0, 2, and 6 months
	Age 15-26	Series of three at 0,2, and 6 months
3. Syphilis screening (mals and females)	When sexually active	PRN or with Pap smear, etc
4. Males:	Adolescence	Monthly
a) Self/Breast/Testicular exams		
5. HIV	Depending on level of sexual activity or IV drug use	Assess knowledge of prevention
6. Tetanus-diphitheria (Td), substitute 1 dose of Tdap for Td	As early as age 7	Every 10 years
7. Meningococcal	All adolescents ages 11-18	Revaccinate x 1 only for high risk
8. Influenza		Annually
9. Pneumococcal (PPSV23)	19-64 if smokes, asthma, COPD, diabetes, alcoholism	
10. PPD screening	Once during adolescence	Every 2 years

YOUNG ADULTS

YOUNG ADULTS(20-39)	When to start?	How often?
1. Complete PE:	Age 20	Every 5 -6 years
2. Females:		
a) Pap smear (with GC and Chlamydia screens)	-Pap age: 21: chlamydia testing for all <25 years of age 21-29 years of age	
I. Cytology (conventional or liquid based)		Every 3 years
II. HPV Co-test	Not to be used for women aged < 30 years old	Every 5 years
b) Self-breast exam	Starting at age 21	Optional
c) Clinical breast exam	Adolescence/now	Every 3 years, annually starting at age 40
d) HPV	Age 9-14	Series of two 6 months apart or series or three at 0, 2, 6 months
	Age 15-26	Series of three at 0,2, and 6 months
3. Males: a) Selfbreast/Testicular exam	Adolescence/now	Monthly
4. HIV	Depending on level of sexual activity or IV drug use	Assess knowledge of prevention
5. BP	Now	With every health care visit or every 2 years
6. Total cholesterol and HDL	Age 20	Every 5 years unless cholesterol> 200 mg/dL
7. Tetanus-disphtheria (Td)	When was last?	Every 10 years
8. Self skin exams	Now	Regularly
9. Influenza		Annually
10. Pneumococcal (PPSV23)	Age 19-64	
11. PPD	Young adult	Controversial but annually for high risk populations
12. Dental cleaning & Checkup	Now	Every 6-12 months

MIDDLE-AGED ADULTS (40-59)	When to start?	How often?
1. Complete PE:	Age 40	Every 5 -6 years
2. Females:		
a) Pap smear (with GC and Chlamydia screens)	-Pap age 21	
I. Cytology (conventional or liquid based)	30-65 years of age	Every 3 years
II. HPV Co-test + HPV test	30-65 years of age	Every 5 years ACOG: Not recommended
b) Self-breast exam	Now	Every year
c) Clinical breast exam	Adolescence/now	
d) Mammography	Beginning at age 40	Every one to 2 years for women ages 40-49, then annually for ages 50-74 or as long as in good health
3. Males:		
a) Selfbreast/Testicular exam	Young adult	Monthly
b) Prostate screening (digital rectal exam and prostate surface antigen (PSA))	• Controversial • Digital exam beginning at age 40 and PSA at age 40 for men with a family history of prostate CA or if African American • All males 50 years of age should have a digital exam and PSA tests	Annually Annually

4. HIV	Depending on level of sexual activity or IV drug use	Assess knowledge of prevention
5. BP	Now	With every health care visit or every 2 years
6. Total cholesterol and HDL	Age 20	Every 5 years unless cholesterol> 200 mg/dL
7. ECG	Age 40	PRN as indicated
8. Colorectal cancer	Age 45	1. Annually fecal occult blood test 2. Flexible sigmoidoscopy q five years 3. Total colon examination by

		colonoscopy every 10 years or by double contrast barium enema every 5-10 years
9. Glaucoma screening	Now	Annually
10. Self skin exam	Now	Regularly
11. Tetanus-diphtheria a) Herpes zoster	When was last? Age 50	Every 10 years Series of two, second dose 2-6 months later
12. Influenza		Annually
13. Pneumococcal	Age 19-64	
14. PPD	Young adult	Controversial but annually for high risk population
15. Dental cleaning & checkup	Now	Every 6-12 months

Middle-aged adults

ELDERLY ADULTS (60 and over)	When to start?	How often?
1. Complete PE: • Laboratory assessments are warranted at this time	Age 60	Every 2 years
2. Females: a) Pap smear (with GC and Chlamydia screens)	-Pap age 21	
I. Cytology (conventional or liquid based)	30-65 years of age	Every 3 years
II. HPV Co-test + HPV test	30-65 years of age	Every 5 years ACOG: Not recommended
b) Self-breast exam	Now	Every year
c) Clinical breast exam	Adolescence/now	
d) Mammography	Beginning at age 40	Every one to 2 years for women ages 40-49, then annually for ages 50-74 or as long as in good health
3. Males: a) Selfbreast/Testicular exam	Young adult	Monthly
b) Prostate screening (digital rectal exam and prostate surface antigen (PSA))	All males> 50 years of age should have a digital exam and PSA test	Annually
4. HIV	Depending on level of sexual activity or IV drug use	Assess knowledge of prevention
5. BP	Now	With every health care visit or every 2 years
6. Total cholesterol and HDL	Age 20	Every 2-5 years unless cholesterol> 200 mg/dL
7. ECG	Age 40	Every 2 years (with cardiac risk factor)
8. Colorectal cancer	Age 45	1. Annually fecal occult blood test 2. Flexible sigmoidoscopy q five years 3. Total colon examination by colonoscopy every 10 years or by double

		contrast barium enema every 5-10 years
9. Glaucoma screening	Now	Annually
10. Self skin exam	Now	Regularly
11. Vaccinations: a) Tetanus-diphtheria b) Influenza vaccine	When was last? Now	Every 10 years Annually
12. Pneumococcal	Age 65 or older	
13. PPD	Young adult	Annually for high risk populations
14. Dental cleaning & Checkup	Now	Every 6-12 months

osteoporosis

- Both sexes experience bone loss with aging
- Osteoporosis in menopause from the loss of estrogen
- In younger women, screen for the female athlete triad:

*Eating disorders, and/or excessive lead to amenorrhea which leads to decreased amounts of estrogen, resulting in bone loss

RISK FACTORS:
1. Early menopause
2. Estrogen deficiency
3. Small frame or underweight
4. Family history
5. High consumption of caffeine, phosphates, protein, sodium
6. Smoking
7. Sedentary lifestyle
8. Alcoholism

TESTING:
1. Dual energy X-ray absorptiometry (DEXA)
- T score compares th patient with the population adjusted for gender, age, and race
- T scores: >-1.0 SD normal
- Between -1.0 to -2.5 is osteopenia
- Below -2.5 is osteoporosis

PREVENTION
- Estrogen replacement therapy
- Avoiding risk factors
- Weight Bearing exercise (30 minutes of exercise 3-5 times a week)
- Calcium intake or supplementation (dairy products, sardines, salmon with bones, green leafy vegetables, tofu, calcium fortified foods)
- Drug therapies: estrogens, bisphosphonates, alendronate, ibandronate, risedronate

PATIENT TEACHING:
- Weight loss
- Fluid management
- Avoid caffeine
- Bladder control strategies
- Pharmacotherapy: muscarinic receptor antagonists:

IMMEDIATE RELEASE

Oxybutynin, Tolterodine, Trospium

EXTENDED RELEASE

Darifenacin, Fesoterodine, Ditropan, Dolifenacin, Detrol LA

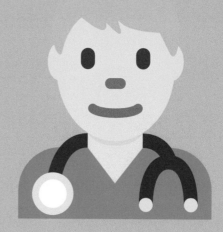

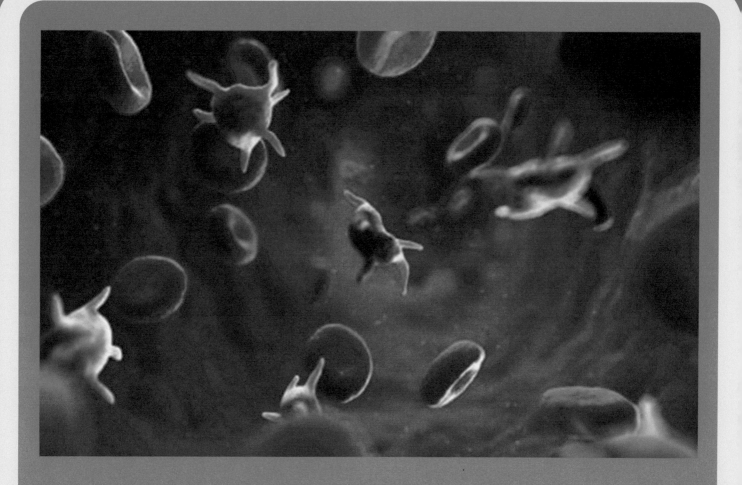

HEMATOLOGICAL DISORDERS

General anemias
Hemophilias
Iron deficiency anemia
Lead poisoning
Leukemias
Sickle cell anemia
Thalassemia

GENERAL ANEMIAS

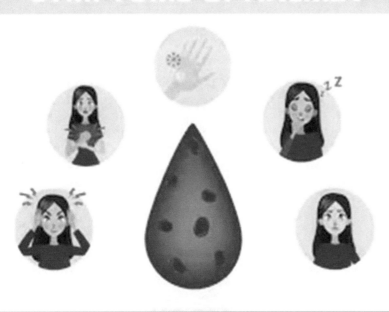

- Microcytic/hypochromic (CHILDREN): IDA, Thalassemia, lead poisoning.

- Normocytic/normochromic: ACD, acute blood loss, early IDA.

- Macrocytic/normochromic (ADULT): Vitamin B12 deficiency, folate deficiency, permicious anemia

HEMOPHILIA A (X-LINKED RECESSIVE)

Deficiency of factor VIII
TYPICAL FINDINGS:
A. Phenotypically normal at birth
B. Bleeding tendency

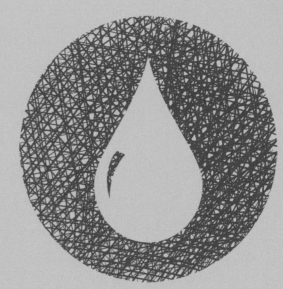

• Microcytic, hypochromic anemia due to a decreased iron intake or slow gastrointestinal blood loss

symptoms

• Fatigue, lethargy, headaches, pica, brittle hair, tachycardia, tachypnea, palpitations, shortness of breath on exertion, delayed motor development, pale, dry skin and mucous membranes, flat, brittle or spoon shaped nails

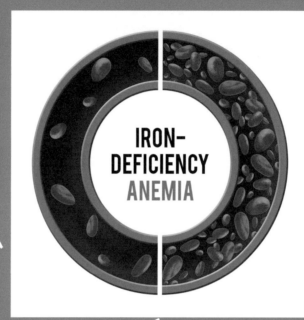

IRON-DEFICIENCY ANEMIA

Laboatory/Diagnostic Findings:

• Hemoglobin and hematocrit low
Low MCV
Low MCHC
Low RBC'S
Increased RDW
Total iron binding capacity (TIBC) increased
Serum Ferritin<30 mg/L
Low serum iron
Reticulocyte count: low in cases of inadequate iron intake, elevated in cases of blood loss

treatment

• 1. Treat with elemental iron 3 to 6 mh/kg/day in one to three doses until hemoglobin normalizes
2. To replace iron stores: 2 to 3 mg/kg/day for four months

LEAD POISONING

Toxic accumulation of leads to iron deficiencies anemia. >5 mg/dl the highest prevalence is among poor, inner-city children, old housing.

SYMPTOMS

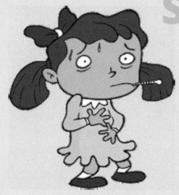

- **VAGUE:**
GI symptoms
SEVERE: lethargy, difficult walking, neuropathies
Headaches
Burtonian lines: bluish discoloration of gingival border
Ataxia
Papilledema

LABORATORY DIAGNOSIS (VENOUS BLOOD LEVEL CONCENTRATION)

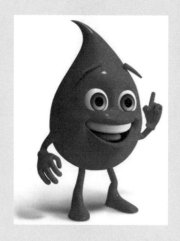

- **Class**
1: Level _< 10 mg/dl
Class IIA: Level 10 to 14 mg/dL (referral to hematologist)
Class IIB: Level 15 to 19 mg/dL
Class III: Level 20 to 44 mg/dL
Class IV: Level 45 to 69 mg/dL (recommend chelation therapy)
Class V: Level <70 mg/dL (hospitalize for chelation, hydration and close observation)

GENERAL TREATMENT

- **Environmental history**
Nutritional history
Physical exam
Oserve
for hemoglobinopathies, impaired renal function, or vitamin D deficiencies.

Leukemias

A group of malignant hematological diseases in which normal
bone marrow elements are replaced by abnormal, poorly
differentiated lymphocytes known as blast cells

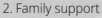

Treatment:
1 Referral to an oncologist
2. Family support

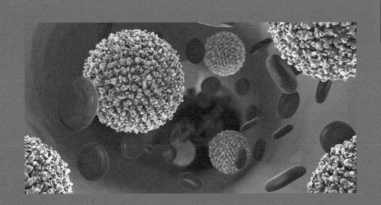

-Anemia
-Pale
-Listless
-Irritable
-Chronically tired
-History of repeated infections
-Bleeding such as epistaxis, petechial, and hematomas
-Lymphadenopathy and hepatosplenomegaly

1. Complete blood count (CBC) with differential WBC, platelet, and reticulocyte counts (thrombocytopenia is present in up to 85% cases, and anemia is usually present)
2. Peripheral smear may demonstrate malignant cells (blasts).
3. Bone marrow will show the poorly differentiated blast cells that have been replacing the healthy bone marrow tissue.

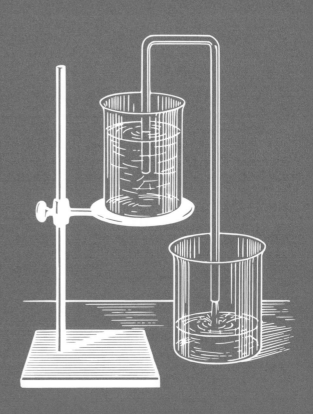

SICKLE CELL ANEMIA

Due to DNA point mutation

1.Autosomal recessive disorder in which Hgb S developes instead or Hgb A
2. Most prevalent in persons of African or African-American ancestry

SYMPTOMS

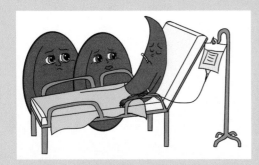

•1.Sickle cell trait (Hgb AS)
a. Usually no clinical symptoms
b. May experience acute painful symptoms under extreme conditions such as
exertion ah high altitudes
2. Sickle cell anemia (Hgb SS)
a. Sudden excrutiatin pain due to a vaso-occlusive crisis usually in the back,
chest, abdomen and long bones
b. Low grade fever
c. Pedisposing factors may be present

TREATMENT

•Collaboration with hematologist
Folic acid supplementation
Immunize with pneumovax (PS-23) and confirm hepatitis B immunity
Provide or refer for genetic counseling
During sickle cell crisis:
Keep client adequately hydrated
Adequate oxygenation
Analgesics for pain control
Antibiotics fo associated infection
Transfuions and/or exchange transfusions for intractable crisis

LABORATORY DIAGNOSTIC FINDINGS

-Hemotocrit 20 to 30°
-Abnormal RBC's
-White blood cells elevated to 12,000 to 15,000
-Indirect biliburbin elevated
-Platelets may be elevated >400,000
-Renal tubular defect

PHYSICAL EXAM FINDINGS

Chronically ill in appearanc Jaundice
Retinopathy
Delayed puberty
Hepatosplenomegaly
Enlarged heart with hiperdynamic precordium
Systolic murmur
Fatigue
Frequent infections

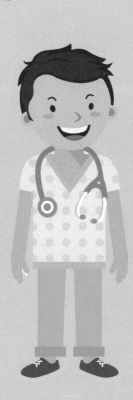

THALASSEMIA

•*A group of hereditary disorders that are characterized by abnormal synthesis of alpha and beta globin chains, caused by autosomal recessive genetic disorder*

SYMPTOMS

•1. Pale or bronze color to skin
2. Tachycardia or tachypnea
3. Hepatosplenomegaly
4. Frontal bossing

PHYSICAL EXAM FINDINGS

•-Prenatal diagnosis
-Newborn screening
-Infancy

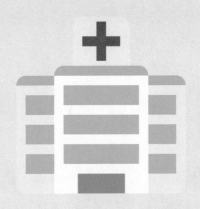

LABORATORY DIAGNOSTIC FINDINGS

•1. CBC
a. HGB
b.MCV
c.Hypochormic RBD's
2. Reticulocyte count
3. Hemoglobin electrophoresis
4. Beta globin gene mapping
5. Ferritin
6.Total bilirubin

INFANCY

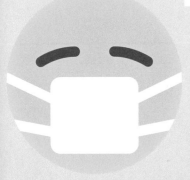

•-FTT/Irritability
-Spelnomegaly
-Pallor/ severe anemia

OLDER CHILD:
-Bony changes
-Splenomegaly
-Iron overload due to multiple transfusion

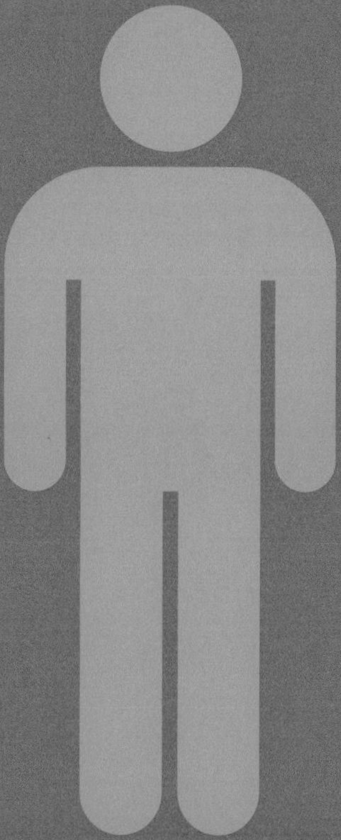

MEN'S HEALTH

-Acute bacterial prostatitis
-Benign prostatic hypertrophy
-Epididymitis
-Erectile dysfunction
-Prostate cancer
-Testicular torsion

acute bacterial prostatitis

Inflammatory infection of the prostate

SYMPTOMS

Fever/chills
Low back pain
Dysuria
Urgency.frequency
Nocturia

PHYSICAL EXAM

Edematous prostate, may be warm and tender/boggy to palpitation, pain

DIAGNOSTIC TESTS

Urine culture-positive for causative agent

TREATMENT

1. Consult/refer if septicemia or urinary retention evident
2. Antibiotic choices:
3. - Single dose ceftriaxone (Rocephin), 250 mg intramuscularly or single dose of cefixime (Suprax) 400 mg orally
4. -Ciprofloxacin 500 mg orally twice daily for 10 to 14 days
5. -Levofloxacin (Levaquin) 500 to 750 mg orally daily for 10 to 1 days
6. 3. Sitz bath three times a day for 30 minutes each treatment

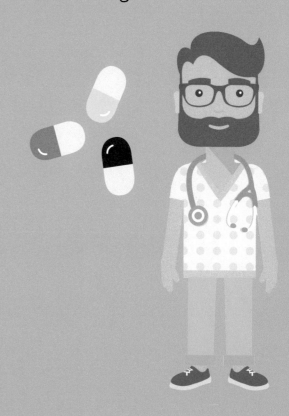

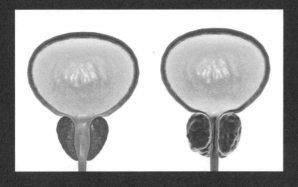

Benign Prostatic Hypertrophy (BPH)

SYMPTOMS

1. Urgency/frequency
2. Nocturia
3. Dribbling
4. Retention

PHYSICAL EXAMINATION

A) Bladder distention may be present
B) Prostate is non-tender with either asymmetrical or symmetrical enlargement
C) Smooth, rubbery consistency with possible nodules

DIAGNOSTICS

-U/A: rules out UTI, no hematuria
-Uroflowmetry
-Abdominal ultrasound: rules out upper tract pathology
-Serum creatinine/ BUN normal
-Prostate-specific antigen (PSA): > 4mg/ml indicates disease
-DRE

TREATMENT

-Observe condition and consult/refer to urologist as needed
-Alpha/blockers: Terazpson (Hytrin), prazosin (Minipress), tamsulosin (Flomax), to relax muscles of the bladder and prostate
-5-alpha-reductase inhibitors: Finasteride (Proscar) and dutasteride (Avodart) to shrink large prostates
-Saw palmetto: effective for some patients

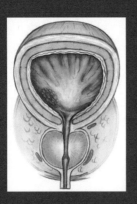

EPIDIDYMITIS

Acute inflammation or infection of the scrotum, secondary to an inflamed epididymis

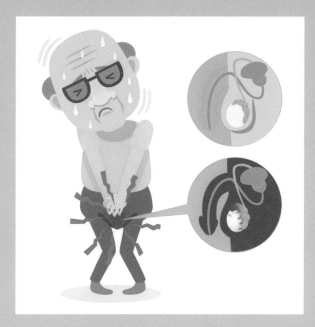

SYMPTOMS

1. Pain
2. Dysuria
3. Urgency/frequency
4. Low back/perineal pain
5. Fever/chills
6. Malaise
7. Scrotal edema

PHYSICAL EXAMINATION

1. Enlarged, tender epididymis
2. Urethral discharge maybe evident
3. Positive Prehn's sign
4. Normal cremasteric reflex, R/O testiculatr torsion

DIAGNOSTIC TEST

1. STD testing
2. Culture of urine
3. Scrotal ultrasound R/O testicular torsion

TREATMENT

1. For acute epididymitis most likely caused by sexually transmitted chamydia and gonorrhea:
2. -Ceftriaxone 250 mg IM in a single dose PLUS
3. - Doxycycline 100 mg orally twice a day for 10 days
4. 2. For acute epididymitis most likely caused by exually transmitted chlamydia and gonorrhea and enteric organisms (men who practice insertive anal sex):
5. -Ceftraxione 250 mg IM in a single dose PLUS
6. -Levofloxacin 500 mg orally once a day for 10 days
7. -Ofloxacin 300 mg orally twice a day for 10 days
8. 3. For acute epididymitis most likely caused by enteric organisms:
9. -Levofloxacin 500 mg orally once daily for 10 days
10. -Ofloxacin 300 mg orally twice a day for 10 days
11. 4. Support/ elevate scrotum
12. 5. Analgesics, NSAID's, ice (early), heat (late), bed rest

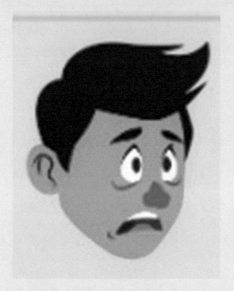

Erectile Dysfunction

Inability to sustain an erection capable of intercourse

MAJOR CAUSES:

Stress:
- Psychosocial issues
- Anxiety (performance)
Atherosclerosis
Diabetes
Recreational drugs:
-Alcohol
-Amphetamines
-Barbiturates
-Cocaine
-Marijuana
-Methadone
-Nicotine
-Opiates

MEDICATIONS (THAT COULD CAUSE ED)

Diuretics
Antihypertensives
H2 blockers
Antidepressants
Anti-anxiety agents
Anti-epileptics
Antihistamines
NSAID's
Muscle relaxants
Parkinson's disease medications

TREATMENT

1. Explore underlying causes
2. Check testosterone level
3. Phosphodiesterase inhibitors> caution with concurrent use of nitrates!
4. - Sildenafil (Viagra)
5. -Vardenafil (Levitra)
6. -Tadalafil (Cialis)
7. -Avanafil

PROSTATE CANCER
Malignant neoplasm of prostate gland

SYMPTOMS

1. Patients are usually asymptomatic
2. May appear to be BPH in early stages
3. In advanced stages: bone pain from metastasis, uremia secondary to obstruction may occur

PHYSICAL EXAMINATION

-Adenopathy
-Bladder distention
-Prostate palpates harder than normal with obscure boundaries, and nodules may be present

LABORATORY/ DIAGNOSTICS

1. Prostate-specific antigen (PSA) values >4 mg/ml = abnormal/ age-specific ranges are based on having/had a PSA <4 mg/ml:

	AGE	VALUE
2.	AGE	VALUE
3.	40-49	<2.5
4.	50-59	<3.5
5.	60-69	<4,5
6.	70-79	<6.5

7. *Thus, the higher the PSA value, the more likely the diagnosis of cancer
8. **Approximately 40% of patients with prostate cancer present with normal PSA values
9. 2. Needle biopsy of prostate
10. 3. Ultrasound to identify solid nodules

TREATMENT

1. Consult/refer
2. Older treatment options: Surgery, radiation, and hormone therapy

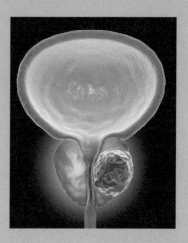

TESTICULAR TORSION

SYMPTOMS

-Sudden onset of testicular pain: may occur after vigorous exercise or testicular trauma
-Nausea, vomiting
-Testicular swelling
-Absent ipsilateral cremasteric reflex!
-Tender, high-riding testicle

TREATMENT

-Immediate urological referral for correction (must correct in <4-6 hours/ irreversible damage after 12 hours)
-Duration of torsion determines if testicle remains viable

MOOD DISORDERS

Anxiety
Bipolar disorder
Depression
Insomnia
Obsessive-compulsive
disorder
PTSD
Squizophrenia
Suicidal ideation

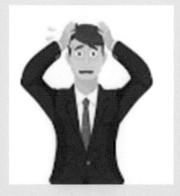

ANXIETY

1st Line Treatment Psychotherapy: cognitive therapy

1st Line Treatment Pharmacology: SSRI and SNRI

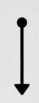

FDA APPROVED:

-Venlafaxine XR   75-225 qd
   -Duloxetine   60 mg qd,
max 120 mg/day; 7-17 yo 30-60 qd, max 120
   -Paroxetine   20
qAM, max 50 mg/day, max elderly 40mg/day,
   -Escitalopram   10 mg qd, max 20
mg/day, max elderly 10 mg/day

NOT FDA APPROVED:

•-Sertraline   50-200 qd
-Fluoxetine   20-80 qd

COMPLEMENTARY AND ALTERNATIVE TREATMENTS

2nd Line Treatment Pharmacotherapy:

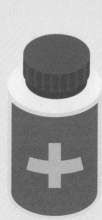

Benzodiazepines:
 Diazepam 2-10 mg bid-qid
 Alprazolam 0.25-0.5 tid, max 4 mg/day; elderly start 0.25 bid-tid
 Lorazepam 2-6 divided bid-tid, max 10 mg/day; elderly start 1-2 mg bid-tid
 Clonazepam 0.25-0.5 bid-tid, max 4 mg/day
 Buspirone 20-30 divided bid-tid, max 60 mg/day; 6-17 yo 15-60 divided bid, max 60

NOT FDA APPROVED:

Venlafaxine XR (6-17 yo) 37.5-225 mg

Augmentation Agents
   Olanzapine   5-10 mg qd
   Risperidone   0.5-1.5 mg qd
   Quetiapine   see above
   Pregabalin   see above

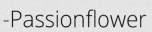

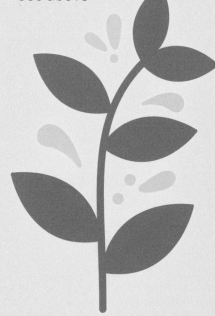

-Passionflower
-Kava
-Valerian
-Theanine

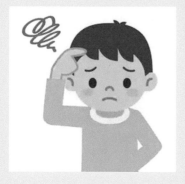

1st Line Treatment Psychotherapy: Cognitive-behavioral therapy for children (CBT)

1st Line Treatment Pharmacology

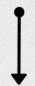

FDA APPROVED:

Sertraline (5-17)
· 25-150 mg qd children 12 and under
· 50-200 mg qd adolescents 13-17
Fluvoxamine (6-17 yo) max 300 mg qd
Fluoxetine (7-17 yo) 10-60 mg qd

NOT FDA APPROVED

Duloxetine (7 to 17 yo)
30-60 mg PO qd; start: 30 mg PO qd x2wk; max: 120 mg/day; may incr. dose in 30 mg increments

2nd Line Treatment Pharmacotherapy

NOT FDA APPROVED

Venlafaxine XR (6-17 yo) 37.5-225 mg

N O T E: These medications were approved for the treatment of anxiety in children before DSM-III and the introduction of the GAD category. They should be considered third-line treatment.

OTHER MEDICATIONS

Diazepam: 1-2.5 mg tid-qid initially, increase gradually as needed and tolerated
Hydroxyzine: < 6 yo 12.5 mg q6-8h; >6 yo 12.5-25 mg q6-8h

DEPRESSION

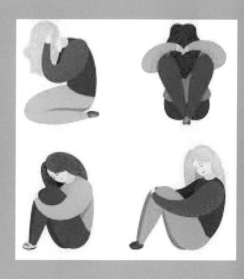

LAB STUDIES TO RULE OUT OTHER ETIOLOGIES

,CBC, chemistry panel, TSH
-Consider FBG, B12, folate (older adults, chronic med history)
-Pregnancy test
-Urine drug screens for substance use disorders
-Others as guided by history, ROS, etc.

1ST LINE TREATMENT PHARMACOTHERAPY:

Antidepressant should be personalized according to clinical findings.

SSRI´S
Celexa
Lexapro
Luvox
Prozac
Zoloft

SNRI´S
Cymbalta
Serzone
Effexor

1ST LINE TREATMENT PSYCHOTHERAPY:

Cognitive-behavioral therapy (CBT)
Interpersonal psychotherapy (IPT)

2ND LINE TREATMENT PHARMACOTHERAPY:

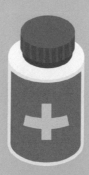

MAOI´S

•-Marplan
•-Nardil
•Parnate

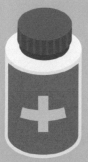

TRYCICLICS

•-Elavil
•-Asendin
•-Anafranil
•-Adapine
•-Sinequan
•-Tofranil
•-Pamelor
•-Vivactil

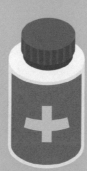

NEWER COMBINATIONS

•-Wellbutrin
•-Norpramin
•-Ludiomil
•-Remeron
•-Desyrel

1ST LINE TREATMENT PSYCHOTHERAPY:

Refer to a counseling psychologist or psychiatrist according on clinical findings.

1ST LINE TREATMENT PHARMACHOTHERAPY:

FDA-approved antidepressants for adolescents:

Fluoxetine and escitalopram
Preadolescents:
fluoxetine

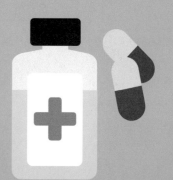

2ND LINE TREATMENT PHARMACHOTHERAPY:

SSRI´S
-Celexa
-Lexapro
-Luvox
-Prozac
-Paxil
-Zoloft

3RD LINE TREATMENT PHARMACHOTHERAPY:

-Venlafaxine
-Duloxetine
-Bupropion
-Mirtazapine

1ST LINE TREATMENT PSYCHOTHERAPY:

Cognitive-behavioral therapy
(CBT)

Interpersonal psychotherapy
(IPT)

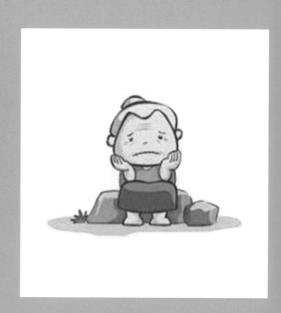

1ST LINE TREATMENT PHARMACHOTHERAPY:

SSRI's, tricyclics and MAOI's. (See table on previous page).

INSOMNIA

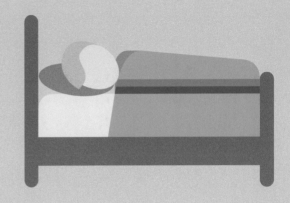

1ST LINE TREATMENT PSYCHOTHERAPY:
COGNITIVE BEHAVIOR THERAPY
(CBT)

MEDICATIONS:

ESZOPICLONE (LUNESTA; GENERAL POPULATION AND OLDER PERSONS)
DOXEPIN (GENERAL POPULATION) HCL 10MG/ML 0.5-1ML AT BEDTIME

RAMELTEON (ROZEREM; OLDER PERSONS)
REMERON (MIRTAZAPINE) 15-45MG QHS
TRAZODONE 25-50MG PO QHS MAX 200/DAY
HYDROXYZINE (NOT FOR ELDERLY)
RESTORIL

OBSESSIVE-COMPULSIVE DISORDER

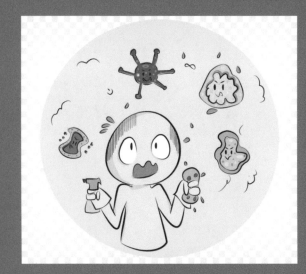

1st Line Treatment Pharmacotherapy:

FDA-approved SSRIs for OCD
Daily (starting FDA max. dose)

Fluoxetine 20-80 mg
Fluvoxamine 50-300 mg
Paroxetine 20-60 mg
Sertraline 50-200 mg

**Not FDA approved
SSRIs for OCD**

Escitalopram 10-20mg
Citalopram 20-40 mg

2nd Line Treatment Pharmacotherapy:

FDA-approved: clomipramine
Not FDA approved: Venlafaxine and Mirtazapine

If partial SSRI response, add clomipramine, antipsychotic, or other agents (e.g., d-amphetamine, memantine, pregabalin, topiramate, lamotrigine, N-acetyl cysteine, clonazepam, lithium, buspirone)

1st Line Treatment Pharmacotherapy (Children):

Daily (starting FDA max. dose)
Fluoxetine 20-60 mg
Fluvoxamine 50-300 mg
Paroxetine 20 to 60 mg
Sertraline 100-200 mg

2nd Line Treatment Pharmacotherapy (Children):

FDA approved SRI for OCD:
Clomipramine
Not FDA approved for OCD:
Venlafaxine, Mirtazapine

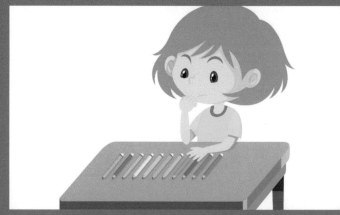

PTSD

1ST LINE TREATMENT PSYCOTHERAPY:

Refer to a counseling psychologist or psychiatrist according on clinical findings.
Cognitive behavioral therapy,
Cognitive processing therapy,
Cognitive therapy.

1ST LINE PHARMACOTHERAPY:

sertraline, paroxetine, fluoxetine and venlafaxine.

SCHIZOPHRENIA

Patient should be refer to counseling, psychologist or Psychiatrist according to clinical findings.

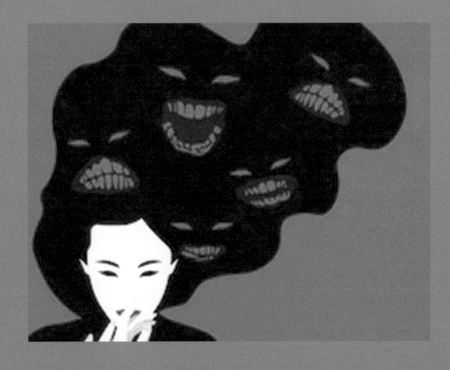

SUICIDAL IDEATION

SUICIDAL RISK FACTORS

- •PRESENCE OF PSYCH DISORDERS
- •HOPELESSNESS
- •IMPULSIVITY
- •HISTORY OF ATTEMPTS

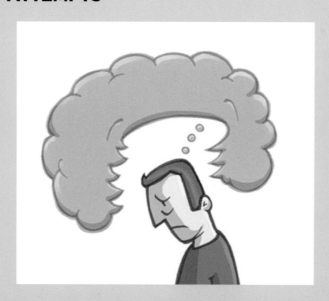

WHAT YOU SHOULD ASK TO THE PATIENT?

- ARE YOU THINKING ABOUT HURTING YOURSELF OR OTHERS? (SUICIDAL IDEATION, HOW LONG?)

- IF YES, DO YOU HAVE A PLAN?
- IF YES, DO YOU HAVE THE MEANS?

IF YES PATIENT NEEDS TO BE REFER FOR INPATIENT EVALUATION AND TREATMENT.

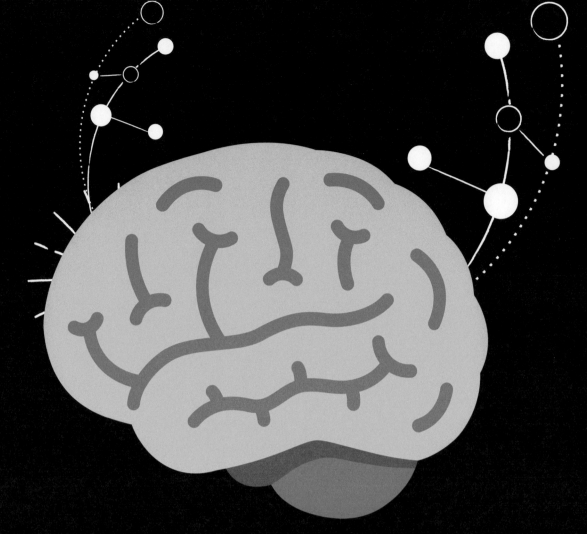

neurological

DISORDERS

ALZHEIMER * BELL'S PALSY * CLUSTER HEADACHES * CRANIAL NERVES * MIGRAINE HEADACHES * MULTIPLE SCLEROSIS * MYASTHENIA GRAVIS * PARKINSON'S DISEASE * SEIZURE * TENSION HEADACHES * TRIGEMINAL NEURALGIA * TRANSIENT ISCHEMIC ATTACK (TIA)

Alzheimer

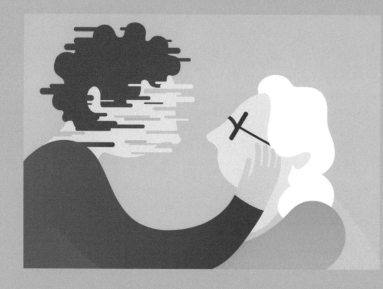

The development of multiple cognitive defects characterized by both memory imapirment (impaired ability to learn new informations and recall previously learned information), and one or more of the following:

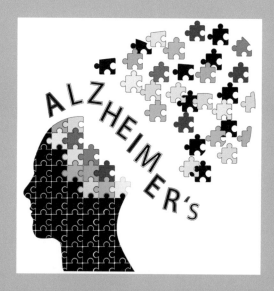

1. *Aphasia (difficulty with speech)*
2. *Apraxia (inhability to perform a previously learned task)*
3. *Agnosia (inability to recognize an object)*
4. *Inability to plan, organize, sequence, and make difference*

DIAGNOSTICS:
-Usual lab diagnostics should be drawn to rule out other diaseases : CBC, lytes, glucose, BUN/CT, LFT's B12, VDRL, etc
-CT to rule out tumors

TREATMENT:
a) Neurological consult
b) Medications to increase the availability of acetylcholine (cholinesterase inhibitors):
- Donepezil (aricept)
- Galantamine (razadyne)
- * Rivastigmine (exelon)
- -Cholinesterase inhibitors are often prescribed in conjuction with NMDA receptor antagonists such as memantine (Namenda) to-decrease symptoms
- c) Refer patient/family for counseling as appropiate

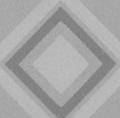

Bell's Palsy

Characterized by a facial paresis, frequently resolving completely without treatment

CAUSES:
-Inflammatory reaction involving the facial nerve
-Idiopathic cause, relationship to reactivation of herpes simplex has been suggested

TREATMENT:
1. Prednisone 60 mg divided in 4 to 5 doses daily and tapered over 7 to 10 days
2. Acyclovir (when facial palsy caused by varicella zoster infection)
3. Lubricating eye drops and patch at night if unable to close
4. Neurology referral as needed

SYMPTOMS:
1. Abrupt onset of facial paresis
2. Pain about the eye may accompany the weakness
3. Face feel stiff and pulled to one side, unable to move forehead
- *Ipsilateral restriction of eye closure*
- *Difficulty with eating and fine facial movements*
- *May be a disturbance of taste*

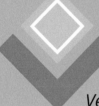

Cluster Headaches

Very painful syndromes, mostly affecting middle-aged men

CAUSES:
-may be precipitated by alcohol ingestion
-Characterized by severe, unilateral, periorbital pain occurring daily for several weeks
-Usually occur at night, awakening the client from sleep
-Usually last less than 2 hours, pain free months or weeks between attacks
-Ipsilateral nasal congestion, rhinorrhea, and eye redness may occur

PHYSICAL EXAM FINDINGS:
The usual exam is normal, may see eye redness and rhinorrhea

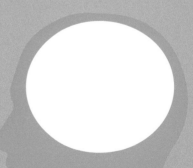

TREATMENT:
Inhalation of 100% O2 may help
Sumatriptan (Imitrex) 6 mg SQ may be effective

cranial nerves

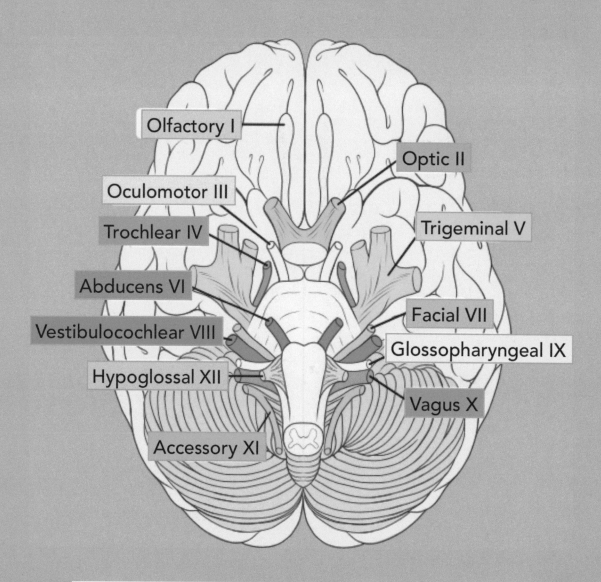

Olfactory I

Optic II

Oculomotor III

Trochlear IV

Trigeminal V

Abducens VI

Vestibulocochlear VIII

Facial VII

Glossopharyngeal IX

Hypoglossal XII

Vagus X

Accessory XI

FUNCTIONS

CN: 1 Smell
CN2: Vision
CN3: Most EOM's, opening eyelids, pupillary constriction
CN4: Down and inward eye movement
CN5: Muscles of mastication, sensation of face, scalp, cornea, mucus membranes and nose
CN6: Lateral eye movement
CN7: Move face, close mouth and eyes, taste (anterior 2/3), saliva and tear secretion
CN8: Hearing and euilibrium
CN9: Phonation, (one-third) gag reflex, carotid reflex, swallowing, taste (posterior)
CN10: Talking, swallowing, general sensation from the carotid body, carotid reflex
CN11: Movement of trapezius and sternomastoid muscles (shrug shoulders)
CN12: Moves the tongue

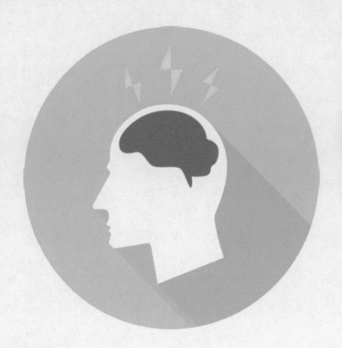

MIGRAINE HEADACHES

MIGRAINE HEADACHES

* *Classic migraine (migraine with aura)*
Common migraine (migraine without aura)
Related to dilation and excessive pulsation of branches of the external carotid artery, typically lasts 2 to 72 hours following the trigeminal nerve pathway

CAUSES:
1. Family history
2. Females more often affected
3. "Triggers' are associated with migraine: emotional or physical stress, lack or excess sleep, missed meals, specific foods, alcoholic beverages, menstruation, use of oral contraceptives
4. Nitrate containing foods
5. Changes in weather

SYMPTOMS:
-Unilateral, lateralized throbbing headache that occur episodically
-May be dull or throbbing
-Gradually and last for several hours or longer
   -Focal neurologic disturbances may procede or accompany migraines
   - Visual disturbances (stars, sparks or zigzag of lights)
   -Aphasia, numbness, tingling, clumsiness, or weakness may occur
   -Nausea and vomiting
   -Photophobia and phonophobia

DIAGNOSTICS:
- Blood chemistries, basic metabolic panel (BMP)
- CBC/ VDRL/ ESR
- CT scan of the head
- Other studies as indicated by the history and physical exam

TREATMENT:
1. Avoidance of trigger factors very important
2. Relaxation/stress manegement techniques
3. Prophylactic daily therapy if attacks occur more than 2 to 3 times per month:
- Amitriptyline (Elavil)
- Divalproex (Depakote)
- Propranolol (Inderal)
- Impramine (Tofranil)
- Clonidine (Catapres)
- Verapamil (Calan)
- Topiramate (Topamax)
- Gabapentin (Neurotin)
- Methysergide (Sansert)
- Magnesium

ACUTE ATTACK:
Rest in dark, quiet room, simple analgesic (ASA), Sumatriptan (Imitrex) 6 mg SQ at onset, may repeat in 1 hour (total of 3 times per day), or 25 mg orally at onset of headache

MULTIPLE SCLEROSIS

CAUSE:
- Autoimmune disease marked by numbness, weakness, loss of muscle coordination, and problems with vision, speech and bladder control
- The body's immune system attacks myelin, a key substance that serves as a nerve insulator and helps in the transmission of nerve signals
--Variable clinical course with remissions and exacerbations

SIGNS/SYMPTOMS:
1. Weakness, numbness, tingling or unsteadiness in a limb, may progress to all limbs
2. Spastic paraparesis
3. Diplopia
4. Disequilibrium
5. Urinary urgency or hesitancy
6. Optic atrophy
7. Nystagmus

DIAGNOSTICS:
- Definitive diagnosis can never be based solely on laboratory findings
- Mild lymphocytosis common
- Slightly elevated protein in CSF
- MRI of the brain

TREATMENT:
1. No treatment to prevent progression of the disease, neurology referral
2. Recovery from acute relapses hastened by steroids, but exent/recovery not improved
3. Antispasmodies
4. Interferon therapy
5. Immunosuppressive therapy
6. Plasmapheresis

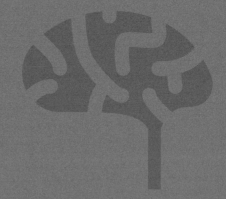

MYASTHENIA GRAVIS

CAUSE:
1. Autoimmune disorder resulting in the reduction of the number of acetylcholine receptor sites at the neuromuscular junction
2. Weakness is typically worse after exercise and better after rest
3. Variable clinical course with remissions and exacerbations

SIGNS/ SYMPTOMS:
- Ptosis
- Diplopia
- Dysarthria
- Dysphagia
- Extremity weakness
- Fatigue
- Respiratory difficulty
- Sensory modalities and DTR's are normal

DIAGNOSTICS:
-Antibodies to acetylcholine receptors (AChR-ab) are found in the serum in = 85% of patients
-Edrophonium (Tensilon) test may be used to differentiate a myasthenic vs cholinergic crisis

TREATMENT:
1. No specific protocol: neurology referral
2. Anticholinestrase drugs block the hydrolysis of acetylcholine and are used for symptomatic improvement
3. Immunosuppressives
4. Plasmapheresis
5. Venilator support may be needed during a crisis

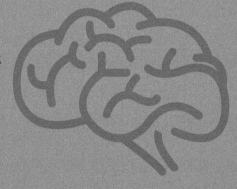

Parkinson's disease

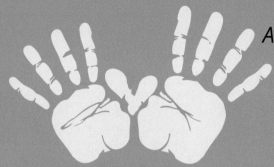

A degenerative disorder as a result of insufficient amount of dopamine in the body

CAUSES:
Onset usually between 45-65 years of age, most commonly is idiopathic

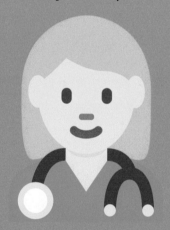

SYMPTOMS:
1. Tremor: slow, most conspicuous at rest, may be enhanced by stress
2. Rigidity
3. Bradykinesia
4. Wooden facies
5. Impaired swallowing
6. Drooling may be observed
7. Decreased blinking
8. Myerson's sign (repetitive tapping over the bridge of the nose produces a sustained blink response)

TRATMENT
1. Increasing available dopamine
- Carbidopa-levodopa (Sinemet)
- Amantadine (symmetrel)
- 2. Anticholinergics helpful in alleviating tremor and rigidity
- Benztropine (cogentin)
- Trihexyphenidyl (artane)
- 3. Others
- Pramipexole (mirapex)
- Ropinirole hydrochoride (requip)

SEIZURE

A variety of paroxysmal events occurring as a result of abnormal electrical activity

1. **Partial (focal, local):**
2. a) Simple partial: common with cerebral lesions
- No loss of consciousness
- Rarely lasts > 1 minute
- b) Complex partial:
- Any simple partial seizure followed by impaired level of conscuousness
- May have aura, staring, or automatisms such as lip smacking and picking at clothing
- **2. Generalized:**
- a) Absence (petite mal): sudden arrest of motor activity with blank stare, begin and end suddenly
- b) Tonic-clonic (grand mal):
- May have an aura
- Begins with tonic contractions (repetitive involuntary contractions of muscle), loss of consciousness, then clonic contractions (maintained involuntary contraction of muscle)
- Usually lasts 2-5 minutes
- **3. Status epilepticus: series of grand mal seizures of > 10 minutes duration**
- a) Medical emergency
- b) May occur when the patient is awake or asleep, but the patient never gains consciousness between attacks
- c) Most life-threatening

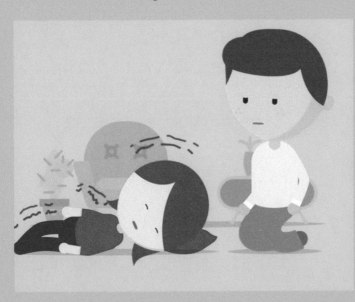

DIAGNOSTICS:
EEG: the most important test in determining seizure classification
CT of the head

TREATMENT:
1. Maintain open airway, protect patient from injuries, administer oxygen if needed
2. Do not force artificial airways or objects between teeth
3. Parenteral benzodiazepines are used to acutely stop seizure activity

SUBSEQUENT SEIZURE PREVENTION:
1. Maintenance doses of long-acting anticonvulsants: carbamezapine (tegretol), ethosuximide (zarontin), phenobarbital (luminal), phenytoin (dilantin), primidone (mysoline), valproic acid (depakene)
2. Additional antiepeleptic drugs: gabapentin (neurontin), lacosamide (vimpat), lamotrigine (lamictal), levetiracetam (keppra), oxcarbazepine (trileptal), pregabalin (lyrica), rufinamide (banzel), tiagabine (gabitril)
3. Dosages should be titrated

Tension headaches

Most common type of headache

HEADACHE
-Location, duration, and quality should be evaluated
-Associated activity: exertion, sleep, tension, relaxation
-Timing of the menstrual cycle
-Associated symptoms
-"Triggers

SYMPTOMS:
1. Vise-like or tight in quality
2. Usually generalized
3. Most intense about the neck or back of the head
4. No associated focal neurological symptoms
5. Last for several hours

TREATMENT:
-Over the counter analgesics
-Relaxation

Trigeminal neuralgia

Nerve disorder that causes a stabbing or electric-shock-like pain in parts of the face

CAUSES:
-Multiple sclerosis
-Pressure on the trigeminal nerve from a swollen blood vessel or tumor

SYMPTOMS:
-Very painful, sharp spasms that last a few seconds or minutes, can become constant
-Pain is usually localized on one side of the face

DIAGNOSTICS:
-Neurological examination
-MRI
-Trigeminal reflex testing

TREATMENT:
1. Anti-seizure drugs
2. Muscle relaxants
3. Tricyclic antidepressants

Transient ischemic attack (TIA)

Periods of acute cerebral insufficiency lasting less than 24 hours without any residual deficits

CAUSES:

-Ischemia due to atherosclerosis, thrombus, arterial occlusion, embolus, intracerebral hemorhage

-Cardio-embolic events (astrial fibrillation, acute MI, endocarditis, valve disease)

-TIA is indicative of an impending stroke

-Approximately 1/3 of patients with TIA will exerience cerebral infarction within 5 years

SYMPTOMS:

1. Altered vision: ipsilateral monocular blindness (amaurosis fugax), homonymous hemianopia (half vision)
2. Altered speech: transient aphasia
3. Motor impairment: paresthesias of contralateral arm, leg, or face
4. Sensory deficits
5. Cognisitve and behavioral abnormalities
6. Dysphagia
7. Vertigo
8. Nystagmus

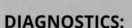

TIA CLASSIFICATIONS:

1. Vertebrobasilar: as result of inadequate blood flow from vertebral arteries: vertigo, ataxia, dizziness, visual field deficits, weakness, confusion, etc.
2. Carotid: due to carotid stenosis, aphasia, dysarthria, altered LOC, weakness, numbness, etc.

DIAGNOSTICS:

-CT is best for distinguishing between ischemia, hemorrhage, and tumor

- MRI is superior to CT in detecting ischemic infarcts

- Echocardiogram

-Carotid doppler/ultrasound

-Cerebral angiography

TREATMENT:

- Aspirin has been shown to reduce the incidence of stroke and death
- Clopidogrel (Plavix) 75 mg/day by mouth
- Asses for hypertension: the #1 cause of heart failure

orthopedic disorders

*ankle sprain
*bursitis
*carpal tunnel syndrome
*costochondritis
*fibromyalgia
*knee injury/pain
*low back pain
*muscle strain
*Morton's neuroma
*osgood-schlatter
*osteoarthritis
plantar fasciitis
*polymyalgia rheumatica
*rheumatoid arthitis
*soft tissue injuries

ankle sprain

CAUSES:

1. **Lateral ankle sprain in the most frequent sports-related injury**

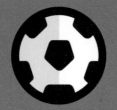

SYMPTOMS:

1. Grade 1: mild, localied tenderness, normal ROM, no disability
2. Grade 2: moderate/ severe pain with weight bearing; difficulty walking, swelling and ecchymosis; pain immediately after injury
3. Grade 3: impossible to ambulate, resist any motion of feet, "egg-shaped-- swelling withing 2 hours of injury

DIAGNOSTICS:

X-rays to rule out fractures
MRI

TREATMENT:

1. R-I-C-E
2. No weight bearing
3. High-dose NSAID's
4. Refer grade 3 sprains for possible casting as needed

bursitis

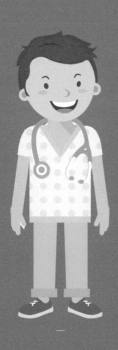

CAUSES:

1. Trauma
2. Sepsis/infection in a joint space
3. Most common locations:
4. -Olecranon
5. -Subdeltoid
6. -Ischial
7. -Perpatellar

DIAGNOSTICS:

1. Aspiration with gram stain and C and S
2. WBC (elevation suggestive of a bacterial infection)
3. Plain x-rays to rule out other bone/joint conditions

SYMPTOMS:

Pain: especially with movement
Swelling
Tenderness
Erythema

TREATMENT:

-Splinting
-R-I-C-E
-Applying heat x 30 minutes TID or QID
-Aspirin or NSAID's
-Steroid injections into bursa
-Is septic: aspiration or I and D with parenteral antibiotics

CARPAL
tunnel syndrome

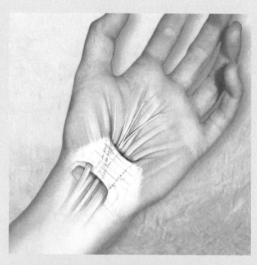

CAUSES:
Idiopathic, associated with repeated wrist flexion

SYMPTOMS:
1. Numbness, tingling, "burning" along the median nerve
2. Nocturnal pain
3. Pain exacerbated with dorsiflexion of wrist
4. Positive Tinel's sign: tapping over the median nerve on the flexor surface of the wrist produces a tingling sensation radiating from the wrist to the hand
5. Positive Phalen's test: reproduction of symptoms after 1 minute of wrist flexion
6. Carpal compression test: pressure with the examiner's thumb over the patient's carpal tunnel for 30 seconds elicits symptoms

DIAGNOSTICS:
Electromyography to document motor involvement
X-rays to rule out other disorders/complications

TREATMENT:
-Elevation, occupational splinting or bracing, NSAID"s, ijection of carpal tunel with corticosteroids, referral for surgical intervention

COSTOCHONDRITIS

INCIDENCE:
Injury
Physical strain
Upper respiratory illness
Infection
Fibromyalgia

SYMPTOMS:
Pain and tenderness where the ribs attach to the breastbone
Pain when taking a deep breath or coughing

DIAGNOSTICS:
Physical exam
X-rays

TREATMENT:
1. Usually resolves on its own
2. Local ice or heat may be helpful
3. NSAID's

fibromyalgia

Widespread muscle pain and tenderness.
Fibromyalgia is often accompanied by fatigue and altered sleep, memory, and mood.
SYMPTOMS MAY INCLUDE
Pain: constant dull body pain that lasts for more than 3 months
Sleep problems
Cognitive difficulty: it is usually referred as fibro fog; difficulties in
focusing or paying attention
Fatigue: people with this condition often feel tired and weak, sleep for longer
periods and wakes up with pain

Causes
Exact cause is not known, it is
believed that the following
are responsible for disease
development:
Genetics: Certain gene mutations
are responsible for this
condition. This tends to run in
the families
Infection: Prior infections can
trigger fibromyalgia and
worsen the symptoms
Physical or emotional trauma:
People with physical or
emotional trauma can develop
this condition
Stress: Stress leaves its effect for
a long time; this can
also be a trigger factor

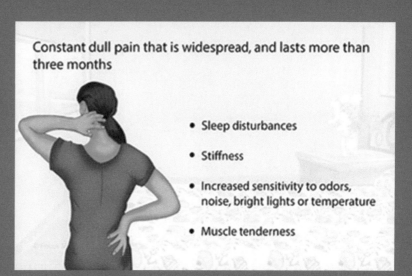

Constant dull pain that is widespread, and lasts more than three months

- Sleep disturbances
- Stiffness
- Increased sensitivity to odors, noise, bright lights or temperature
- Muscle tenderness

Treatment
Treat underlying symptoms
and commorbidities.
Refer patient to
rheumatologist

Prevention
It cannot be prevented.
Medication and lifestyle changes can improve the symptoms.

Complications
May lead to loss of ability to focus and pay attention at
workplace or home.
Pain and Fatigue
Sleep problems
These may also lead to depression.

KNEE INJURY/PAIN

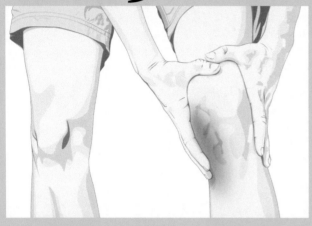

Due to mechanical, inflammatory and/or degenerative problems

CAUSES:
1. Trauma
2. Exercise
3. Medial meniscus tears are 10 x more common than lateral tears

SYMPTOMS:
1. "Locking" usually indicaive of meniscal tear or loose bodies
2. "Giving way"
3. Swelling
4. Crepitus
5. McMurray's test: and audible/palpable click when the lnee is raised slowly with one foot externally rotated (knee is flexed then quickly straightened): NP's hand rests on the joint line, test is positive for medial meniscal injuries
6. Lachman's test> drawer test to asses for anterior/posterior cruciate ligament tear
7. -Most sensitive and easy to perform test on a swollen, painful knee
8. -Place knee in 20-30 minutes degree flexion, gras leg with one hand with anterior force to proximal tibia (stresses the ACL/PCL) while the opposite hand stabilizes the thigh, grades 1+ to 3+ grade of displacement

9. Apley's grind test: flex knee 90 degrees with patient prone, put pressure on heel with one hand while rotatin the lower leg internally and externally, pain or click is positive for medial or lateral collateral ligament damage and/or meniscus injury

DIAGNOSTICS:
Lab examination only inidcated if arthritis is suspected
X-rays of knees AP and lateral
MRI

TREATMENT:
Immobilization/rest (R-I-C-E)
NSAID's
ROM
Aspirate effusions as needed
Consultation-referral

LOW BACK PAIN

Any pain perceived by the patient as originating from the lumbosacral region of the spinal column, may be localized or radiate to the leg and/or feet

COMMON CAUSES:
Mechanical strain, obesity, poor body mechanics, trauma, repetitive twisting, bending or lifting, herniated lumbar disks, lumbar spinal stenosis, other

DIAGNOSTICS:
X-rays AP/lateral films of the spine
CT or MRI

SYMPTOMS:
Pain in low back region, may have radiating pain
Decreased muscle strenght or actual atrophy of muscle

TREATMENT:
1. Functional bracing with orthotic devices
2. Rest, physical therapy
3. Weight loss
4. Utrasound/transcutaneous electric nerve stimulator (TENS)
5. NSAID's
6. Refer

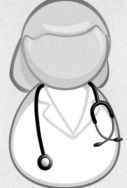

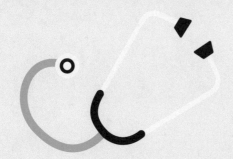

MUSCLE STRAIN

SYMPTOMS:
Pain during ROM
Edema
Ecchymosis

TREATMENT:
R-I-C-E
Assistive devices as needed
Analgesics
NSAID's
Prevention education

Caused by overuse of muscle tendons, often occurring with repetitive movement, resulting in inflammation

Morton's neuroma

A benign neuroma causing a compression neuropathy of an intermetatarsal plantar nerve, most commonly on the 3rd or 4th intermetatarsal spaces

CAUSES:
-Usually injury of the nerve from high-heeled shoes
-High impact activities
-Flatfeet, bunions, and hammertoes may contribute to the problem

SYMPTOMS:
-A feeling as though "standing on a pebble" in the shoe
-Shooting pain affecting the halves of the 2 toes
-Tingling or numbness in the shoes

DIAGNOSTICS:
Ultrasound, MRI for lesion

TREATMENT:
-Orthotics and corticosteroid injections
-Referral for cryogenic neuroablation or neurectomy

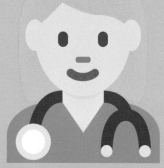

Osgood-Schlatter

Rupture of the growth plate at the tibial tuberosity as a result of stress on the patellar tendon

SYMPTOMS:
-Painful limp with pain below the knee cap
-Swelling ranges from mild to very severe

DIAGNOSTICS:
-Physical exam
-X-ray to rule out other conditions

TREATMENT:
R-I-C-E
NSAID's or acetaminophen
Refer to surgery

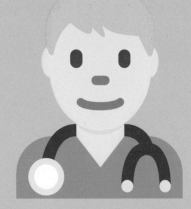

OSTEOARTHRITIS (OA)

Degenerative joint disease with slow destruction of the articular cartilage

Inflammation: Asymmetrical
Age: 53-64 years
Gender: Men & women equally affected
Labs: N/A
Stiffness/Pain: Better in the morning

JOINTS:
-Weight-bearing (knee, hip) + fingers, hands, wrists
-Swelling & edema- but no redness or "heat" complaints to joints
-Heberden's nodes, distal interphalangeal joints (DIPS's)
-Bouchard's nodes, proximal interphalangeal joints (PIP's)

TREATMENT:
ASA
Acetaminophen
NSAID's (Ibuprofen, naproxen)
COX-2 inhibitors celecoxib (celebrex)

X-RAY FINDINGS:
-Narrowing of the joint space
-Osteophytes
-Juxia-articular sclerosis
-Subchondral bone

DIAGNOSTICS:
Synovial aspirate normal, clear/yellow

SUPPORTIVE CARE:
-Weight loss
-Use canes on opposite side
-Ice (improve ROM)
-Moist heat (decrease muscle spasms and relieve stiffness)
-Physical therapy
-Refer for joint replacement

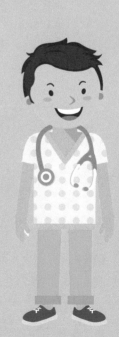

PLANTAR FASCIITIS

Inflammation of plantar fascia, the thick tissue on the bottom of the foot that connects the heel bone to the toes and creates the arch of the foot

CAUSES:
-Foot arch pain/problems
-Obesity, sudden weight gain
-Particularly common in runners

SYMPTOMS:
- Pain and stiffness in the bottom of the heel
*Heel pain may be dull or sharp, radiates from the heel to the toes
*The bottom of the foot may also ache or burn
*Pain is worse in the morning or after standing for awhile

DIAGNOSTICS:
-Physical exam
- X-rays taken to rule out other problems

TREATMENT:
Medications (NSAID's, corticosteroids)
Orthotics
Night splints
Physical therapy
Referral for surgery

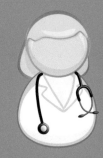

POLYMYALGIA RHEUMATICA

An inflammatory disorder involving pain and stiffness in the shoulder and, usually, the hip

CAUSES:
-Etiology is unknown
-Almost always occurs in people over 50 years

SYMPTOMS:
-Stiffness in neck, shoulders, and hips
-Loss of range of motion in affected areas
-Fatigue, anemia, and mild fever

DIAGNOSTICS:
-Erythrocyte sedimentation rate (ESR)
-X-rays as needed to rule out other conditions

TREATMENT:
-Corticosteroids
-Symptomatic management

Rheumatoid Arthritis (RA)

Rheumatoid Arthritis (RA)

Systemic autoimmune disease-causing inflammation of connecitve tissue

Inflammation: Symmetrical
Age: 35-50 years
Gender: Women more common (3:1)
Labs: ESR usually elevated, ANA (+) in 1/5 patients
Stiffness/Pain: Worse in the morning

JOINTS:
-Proximal interphalangeal joints (PIP's)
-Metacarpophalangeal joints (MCP's)
-Wrists
-Swelling & edema with redness and "heat" complaints to joints

DIAGNOSTICS:
-Synovial aspirate with inflammatory changes and WBC's

TREATMENT:
-High dose salicylates
-NSAID's
-Disease modifying antirheumatic drugs (DMARDS):
*Corticosteroids
*Methotrexate
*Antimalarials (hydroxychloroquine)
*Gold salts injections

X-RAY FINDINGS:;
-Joint swelling
-Progressive cortical thinning
-Osteopenia
-Joint space narrowing

SUPPORTIVE CARE:
-Early rheumatologist referral
-Rest
-Physical therapy
-Surgery

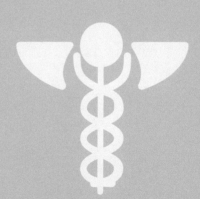

soft tissue
INJURIES

Injury that occurs in non-osseous structures of the musculoskeletal system, such as muscles, bursa, fibrous connective tissue that connects muscle to bone, or cartilage (dense conncective tissue with no blood supply)

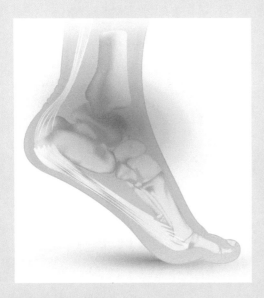

CLASSIFICATION OF INJURIES:
1. Abrasions
2. Contusions
3. Hematomas
4. Lacerations/tears
5. Strains
6. Sprains

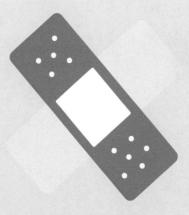

TREATMENT:
1. R-I-C-E of injured par
2. Immobilization may be necessary, dependent on location, severity, and type of injury:
3. *Casts
4. *Splints
5. *Immobilizers
6. *Slings
7. 3. Pharmacologic interventions:
8. -NSAID's for mild to moderately severe injuries:
9. *Ibuprofen 400 to 800 mg TID to QID
10. *Naproxen 250 to 500 mg every day in divided doses
11. 4. Physical therapy
12. 5. Referral

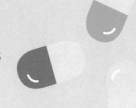

OBSTETRIC &

PREGNANCY

ABORTION

Pregnancy termination at any time prior to viability (24 weeks) through spontaneous exoulsion or medical/surgical removal.

- Approximately 15% of pregnancies will abort spontaneously in the first trimester
- Losses in the 2nd trimester are due to cervical incompetence, infection, or uterine abnormalities

SYMPTOMS:
- Vaginal bleeding of varying degrees
- Cramping/pelvic pressure
- Low back pain
- Rupture of membranes
- Hemodynamic changes in vital signs of hemorrhage is involved

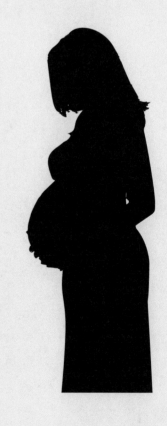

DIAGNOSTIC TESTS (SPONTANEOUS AB):
-hCG levels
-Ultrasound
-CBC, type, and Rh
-Coagulation profile as needed

TREATMENT (SPONTANEOUS AB):
-Refer
-Bed rest if threatened, inevitable
-Abstinence
-Labs

TREATMENT (INDUCED OR ELECTIVE AB):
1. *Surgical Abortion*
- Vaccum D and C: to 12 weeks
- D and E: 13 to 14 weeks to 29 to 22 weeks
- Hysterotomy/hysterectomy
2. *Medical: indicated through 49 days pregnancy*
- Mifepristone (Mifeprex)
- Prostagladin (Misoprostol)

ABRUPTO PLACENTAE

ABRUPTO PLACENTAE

Separation of the placenta from the uterine wall, comletely or partially

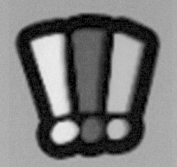

- Complete abruption is an abtetrical emergency and unless hospitalized at the time of the event, fetal death is very likely
- Abruption usually occurs in the second or third trimesters and may be initiated by a number of factors
- Hemorrhage may be sudden and life threatening to the mother

SYMPTOMS:

- Severe abdominal pain
- Bright red bleeding is heavy if unconcealed
- May be minimal to moderate bleeding if abruption is concealed
- Uterus is rigid in concealed abruption
- Shock
- Fetal distress/absent FHT's

TESTS:

1. Ultrasound to locate placental implantation
2. EFM to monitor for fetal distress
3. CBC, type, and Rh for transfusion, coagulation profiles to monitor hemodynamic changes

TREATMENT:

1. Immediate transport and referral: physician management
2. If hemorrhage and/or fetal distress are present, immediate delivery when mother becomes stable

COMPLICATIONS OF
PREGNANCY

HYPERTENSIVE DISORDERS

1. Pregnancy induced hypertension (PIH): BP> 140/90, or rise in systolic >30 mmHg or diastolic > mmHg above an established baseline on at least 2 occasions, with readings six hours apart
2. Preeclampsia: PIH + proteinuria + generalized edema after 20 weeks gestation
3. Eclampsia: preeclampsia + seizure activity
4. HELLP syndrome: **H**emolysis **E**levated **L**iver enzymes and a **L**ow **P**alatelet count

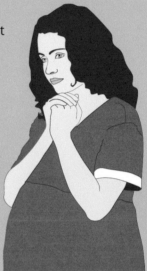

PIH

PREDISPOSING FACTORS:
- Pre-existing hypertension, renal, cardiovascular disease
- Diabetes
- Lupus
- Multiple gestation
- Primigravida
- Personal or family history of PIH, preeclampsia
- Maternal age at either en of reproductive time line

TESTING:
- BP surveillance
- CBC, LFT's, 24 hour urine for protein, creatinine/creatinine clearance
- NST after 32 to 34 weeks or PRN
- Ultrasound PRN, usually for lag in fetal growth as a result of PIH

TREATMENT:
- Rest at home: if condition worsens, bed rest in left lateral recumbent position
- Fetal surveillance: NST, ultrasound, and kick counts for fetal activity at home

PREECLAMPSIA

SYMPTOMS:
- Sudden weight gain
- Progression from digital and mild facial edema to generalized edema
- Frontal or occipital headaches
- Visual disturbances

PHYSICAL FINDINGS:
1. Hypertension
a) > 140/90 mm Hg or ? 30/15 mm Hg above established baseline
2. Proteinuria
a) Trace to +1 on a voided sample, progressin to +2 with worsening condition
3. Edema
a) Nondependent edema > 1+ progressing to pretibial edema > 3 to 4 +
b) Worsening facial and generalized edema
4. Weight gain
a) Greater than 2 pounds per week or 6 pounds in one month
b) Lagging fundal height
5. Reflexes
a) WNL progressing to 3-4 + with worsening condition

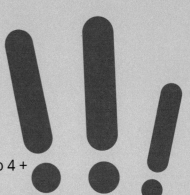

TESTING:
1. Bp surveillance
2. Urine testing every visit, repeat 24 hour urine testing PRN
3. Baseline labs . Coagulation studiesnwith worsening condition
4. NST weekly, biphysical profile (amnionic fluid index must be included)
5. Ultrasound to monitor fetal growth and evaluate placetal condition PRN

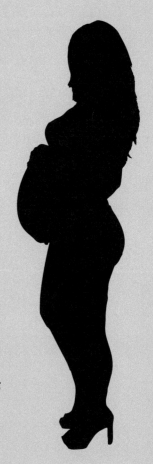

TREATMENT:
-Referral
-Strict bed rest with worsening condition in left lateral recumbent position
-Fetal surveillance: NST, BPP, ultrasound
-Kick count at home
-Weekly steroid injection (B-methasone) for fetal lung maturity if <34 weeks gestation
Hospitalization and MgSO4 therapy to stabilize if severe condition, then delivery if fetal maturity assured (> 34 weeks or 2 doses of B-methasone)

ECLAMPSIA

SYMPTOMS:
1. PIH + pre-eclampsia + Seizure
2. May have prodromal symptoms of

a) severe headache

b) Epigastric or RUQ pain wich progressively or suddenly worsens

c) Visual changes, including spotty vision, blurriness, blindness

3. BP consistently elevated above 160/100
4. Tonic-clonic seizures
5. Oliguria, may progress to anuria
6. Fetal distress in utero (FDIU)

TESTING:
- CBC, LFT's with full chemistry profile, coagulation profile, 24 hour urine for protein, creatinine/creatinine clearance, uric acid
- Fetal surveillance continous in hospital

TREATMENT:
- Refer physician management
- MgSO4 to break seizure (valium if ineffective) then IV drip to stabilize
- Anticipate delivery as soon as stable

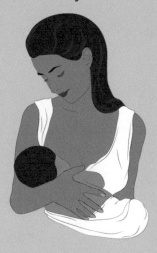

HEMOLYSIS, ELEVATED LIVER ENZYMES AND LOW PLATELETS (HELLP) SYNDROME

SYMPTOMS:
1. Those of preeclampsia
2. Nausea, with or without vomiting
3. Jaundice
4. Extreme fatigue, ill-feeling

PHYSICAL FINDINGS:
- Hepatomegaly
- Tenderness or pain in RUQ, extending to epigastric area
- Jaundice
- Possible ascites

TESTS:
- Thrombocytopenia, below 50,000 not unusual
- Clotting factors reduced
- Severe hemoconcentration
- Very elevated LFT's
- Proteinuria consisten with severe preeclampsia

TREATMENT:
- Refer
- Hospitalization
- Delivery as soon as stable

Contraceptive Options

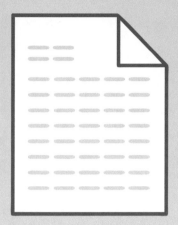

Combined Hormonal Contraceptives (CHC's): the pill, the ring, and the patch. Contain estrogen and progestin, although the combinations vary by product

Short-acting Hormonal Methods

Oral Contraceptives Pills:

CATEGORIES:
1. Combination
- Conventional packs:
A) Usually contain 21 active and 7 inactive pills or 24 active and 4 inactive pills
B) Bleeding occurs when the patient takes the inactive pills
- Continous dosing or extended cycle packs:
A) Usually contain 84 active and 7 inactive pills
B) Bleeding usually occurs only 4 times each year when the inactive pills are taken
- Other formulations: (levonorgestrel/ethinyl estradiol (amethyst)): 365-day continuous pill-contains no inactive pills and bleeding will not occur for the entire year
2. Minipill: contains inly progestin. Thickens the cervical mucus and the endometrium, most likely changing tubal transport of the oocyte and sperm

ADVANTAGES:
- Decreased menstrual cramps and pin
- Less menstrual blood flow
- Improvement in facial acne
- May provide protection against ovarian and endometrial cancer, ectopic pregnancy, pelvic inflammatory disease (PID), functional ovarian cysts, endometriosis, uterine fibroids, among others

DISADVENTAGES:
- May lead to mood changes
- Increased risk of rare liver tumors
- Possible side effects sucha as nausea, headaches, breakthrough bleeding

CONTRAINDICATIONS:
- History of thromboembolic disorders
- CVA (history of)
- Coronary artery disease (CAD)
- Known or suspected breast carcinoma
- Known or suspected estrogen-dependent neoplasia
- Pregnancy
- Bening or malignant liver tumor
- Previous cholelithiasis during pregnancy
- Undiagnosed, abnormal uterine bleeding

TREATMENT:
1. General considerations:
- Begin with low-dose combined or multiphasic pill (35 mcg or less)
- Progestin-only pills may be used in women with history of migraine headaches, who are breast feeding or who have some contraindication to combination pills

2. Adverse effect:
- Abnormal menstrual bleeding: breakthrough bleeding and spotting ay be common, may need a higher dose
- Amenorrhea or hyperenorrhea: often caused by low amount of pprogestin. May need dose increased
- Birth defects: estrogen= pregnancy category X. Immediately discontinue oran contraceptives if pregnant
- Cancer: estrogens promote certain types of breast cancer, patients with + breast CA family history should not take OC's
- Hypertension: risk is increased with afe, dose, and length of therapy
- Weight pain, increased appetite, fatigue, depression, acne, and hirsutism: often caused by high amounts of progestin, may need lower dose
- Nausea, edema, and breast tenderness: caused by high amounts ofestrogen. May need lower dose
- Thromoembolic disorders: increased risk in some patients. OC's contraindicated in patients with a history of thromboembolic disorders, CVA, CAD, or heavy smokers
- Drug-drug interactions: certain antibiotics and anticonvulsants low the effectiveness of OC's

Nuva Ring:

Flexible, prescriptive contraceptive ring, approximately 2 inch in diameter, for the purpose of preventing pregnancy. Effectiveness 92 to 99.7 %

How it works?

Releases synthetic estrogen and progestin, providing pregnancy protection for 1 month.
Release of hormones is activated by vaginal contact.
Prevents ovulation, thickens the cervical mucus, inhibiting sperm penetration.

PROS

- Once per month
- Easily reversible
- Fewer mood swings reported than with oral contraceptives
- May lead to shorter, lighter, and more regular menstrual periods
- Decreased menstrual cramps, improvement of facial acne, depression

CONS

- Breast tenderness, headaches, weight gain, nausea, mood changes, breakthrough bleeding
- Increased vaginal discharge, irritation, or infection
- Diaphragms, cervical caps, or shields cannot be used as a back-up method of contraception while using the ring
- May worsen depression in patients previously diagnosed
- No protection from HIV/AIDS or STD's/STI's

Contraindications

- Age> 35 years
- Smoking
- Uncontrolled high blood pressure
- History of blood clots or any cardioembolic disorder
- Others

How to use?

1. Vaginally inserted one time a month
2. The ring is left in place for 21 days
3. The ring is removed by the patient
4. A new ring must be inserted on the same day of the week as it was inserted in the last cycle or pregnancy may occur
5. If the ring slides out it must be reinserted within 3 hours

The Patch:

Transdermal contraceptive patch that releases synthetic estrogen and progestin.
Failure rate: <1 to 2%

How it works?

Primarly prevents ovulation

PROS

- Once per week
- Could be worn for three weeks
- Easily reversible

CONS

- Site reactions
- SImilar to OC's such as breast tenderness
- No protection from HIV/AIDS
- Reduced effectiveness in women > 90 kg

Contraindications

- Age > 35 years
- Smoking
- High blood pressure
- History of blood clots or any cardioembolic disorder
- Others

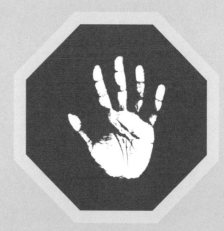

How to use?

1. First patch is applied to the arm, buttocks, torso, or abdomen o either the first day of her menstrual cycle or on the first Sunday following that day, whichever is preferred
2. The patch is removed seven days later, and another patch is applied
3. 1 patch/7 day period x 3 patches, then 7 days without a patch, then start again.
4. If the patch stays off for > 24 hours, restarting a new 4 week cycle is necessary, along with using a backup method of contraception

Injected Contraception:

Depo-Provera (DMPA) Long-acting progestin administered by intramuscular injection to prevent pregnancy and/or provide hormonal control of the menstrual cycle. Failure rate < 1%

How it works?

- Suppresses follicle-stimulating hormone (FSH) and luteinizing hormone (LH), thus blocking the LH surge, which will inhibit ovulation
- Thickness cervical mucus
- Alters the endometrium by creating a thin, atrophic lining

PROS

- Highly effective, long acting, convenient
- Decreased anemia, cramps, ovulatory pain
- Useful in reducing pain associated with endometriosis
- Possible reduction in risk of PID and endometrial and ovarian cancers

CONS

- Menstrual irregularities
- Delayed return of fertility (up to 1 year)
- Injection every 3 months
- Possible reduction in bone density with long-term use

Contraindications

- Allergy to DMPA
- Unexplained abnormal uterine bleeding
- Pregnancy

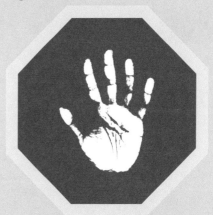

How to use?

1. Pregnancy test if greater than 2 weeks since 3 month period ended
2. Injection is given intramuscular every 3 months with 2 week grace period
3. Backup method should be used during the first 2 weeks after the injection, unless administered by DOC 5

Implant contraception:

Nexplanon, a single and thin, flexible rod which contains etonogestrel and releases low diffusion of progestin from the rod.

How it works?

Same as other progestins, long-acting reversible contraceptive

PROS

- Continuous protection for 3 years
- No estrogen related side effects
- Lowered or absent menses/decreased anemia
- May low risk of endometrial cancer

CONS

- Requires informed consent
- Irregular menstrual periods, including prolonged menses, spotting between periods, absent periods
- Implant may be slightly visible initially

Intrauterine Device (IUD):

An artificial device with either a metal wrapping or chemically-impregnated surface.
Failure rate: 1 to 3.0%

TYPES

1. Hormonal: progestin-releasing (Mirena)= T-shaped plastic device, can remain in the uterus from 3 to 6 years depending on the product
2. Non-hormonal: Copper (ParaGard)= T-shaped plastic decive wrapped with fine copper wire, can remain in the uterus up to 10 years

How it works?

1. Immobilizes sperm and interferes with migration of sperm from the vagina to the fallopian tubes
2. Speeds transport of the ovum through the fallopian tube
3. Inhibits fertilization
4. Causes lysis of the blastocyst and/or prevents implantation due to local foreign body inflammatory responses

PROS

- Progestin-releasing IUD's may decrease menstrual loss and dysmenorrhea
- Can prevent Asherman's Syndrome

CONS

- Pain and cramping may occur
- Increase in menstrual nleeding resulting in anemia
- If pregnancy already occur:
*Spontaneous abortion in up to 50% cases if IUD left in uterus
*Ectopic prgnancies occur in 5% of users

Contraindications

- Active, recent or recurrent pelvin infection, including GC and chlamydia
- Pregnancy
- Risk for PID
- Abnormal uterine bleeding

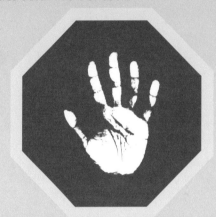

How to use?

1. Requires informed consent
2. May be inserted anytime during cycle, expulsion greater durng menses
3. May insert 4 to 8 weeks postpartum
4. Check, string, monitor bleeding, pain control
5. Danger signs (menses late, abdominal pain or dyspareunia, fever, chills

Barrier Methods:

Flexible, dome-shaped cup constructed of latex rubber works by blocking the transport of sperm through the cervical os. Failure rate: =18%

How it works?

Barrier against sperm transport, when used with spermicidal cream or gel, destroys the cell membrane of the sperm

PROS

- May provide some protection against STD's when used with spermicidal gel
- Relatively safe and easy to use
- Provides immediate protection

CONS

- Skin irritations may occur secondary to latex or spermicide
- Possible increased risk of urinary tract infections and vuvlovaginitis

How to use?

1. Should check for holes, tears periodically
2. Should have diaphragm refitted if weight gain exceeds 20 lbs
3. Avoid oil-based lubricants
4. Must be left in vagina for at least 6 hours following intercourse
5. Must instill spermicide in vagina (nor removing diaphragm) for repeated intercourse

Spermicides:
Preparations which contain chemicals, nonoxynol-9 or octoxynol, whose purpose is to destroy sperm cells. Failure rate 21%

PROS

- Purchased over-the-counter (OTC)
- Relatively safe
- Enhances effectiveness of barrier methods

CONS

- May cause vaginal or penile skin irritation
- Suppositories may dissolve incompletely
- Unpleasant taste

Condoms:
Sheath-like covering usually made of latex which is inserted over the penis or into the vagina. Failure rate: Male 12% Female 21%

PROS

- Purchased OTC
- Relatively safe
- Provides immediate protection against pregnancy and transmission of most STD's

CONS

- May produce less sensation
- Condoms could tear or slip
- Foreplay is interrupted
- If natural skin condoms are used, there is no protection against STD's

How to use?

1. Avoid use of oil-based lubricants
2. Lubrication will increase sensation
3. Reduce risk of condom breakage: leave 1/2 inch of empty pace at end of condom
4. Effectiveness is increased if used with spermicide

Emergency Contraception:

Mechanism used to either prevent fertilization or the implantation of a fertilized egg in the uterus

TYPES:

1. Oral contraception> may be taken within 120 hours (5 days) of unprotected sex
- Levonorgestrel (Plan B- One step, take action, my way, after pill, others). Effectiveness 89% or better if taken within 72 hours
- Over the counter, nonprescription
-Work best if taken within 72 hours (3 days) after unprotected sex
-One should stress that this is not the abortion pill
2. Intruterine devide (IUD): used up to 120 hours (5 days) after unprotected sex
- Copper IUD (Paragard): most effective type of emergency contraception. Effectiveness 99% or better.

PROS

- Avoid unwanted pregnancy

CONS

- Nausea
- Headaches
- Changes in the patient's next menstrual period
- Breast tnderness
- Fluid retencion
- Dizziness
- Diarrhea

Sterilization:

Surgical procedure which interrupts either the fallopian tube or the vas deferens to prevent the passage of oocytes and sperm
Failure rate Female 1: 400 Male 1: 600

How it works?

- Female tubal occlusion
- Male vasectomy

PROS

- Permanent form of contraception for both male and female
- Failure rates are low

Contraindications

Indecision regarding future childbearing

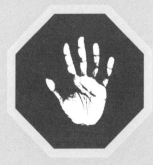

Fertility Awareness Methods/Natural Family Planning:

Planned abstinence from sexual intercourse during that phase of the menstrual cycle when fertility is optimal, with the purpose of preventing pregnancy and enhancing the planning of family.
Failure rate: 20%

How it works?

- *Calendar method/rhythm method:*
a) Record serial cycles, indentifying longest and shortes cycles
b) Determine fertile phase by subtractin 18 days from the shortest cycle and 11 days from the longest cycle
c) Abstain during this time frame
- *Basal body temperature graph:*
a) Record daily bbt prior to rising in AM over a 3 to 4 month period
b) Temperature drops 12-24 hours prior to ovulation, rises following ovulation due to production of progesterone
c) Avoid intercourse from 2 to 3 days prior to expected drop to approximately 3 days following the rise
- *Cervical mucus test:*
a) Record changes in cervical mucus over 3 to 4 month period
b) Notice when mucus changes from scant and thick amounts to thin, with increasing Spinnbarkeit
c) Abstain from time of mucus change until approximately 4 days after change
- *TwoDay method*: variation of the cervical mucous test
a) Check cervical mucus at least twice each day
b) To prevent pregnancy, avois sexual intercourse or use a barrier methods of contraception
- *Symptothermal method:* method that used both the basal ody temperature and cervical mucus techniques
- *Lactational amenorrhea method:* patient relies on breastfeeding for natural family planning, as breastfeeding often delays the onset of ovulation and menstruation for approximately 6 months

CONS

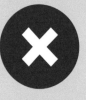

- Pregnancy
- No protection against HIV/AIDS or STD's/STI's
- Some methods limit sexual activity for approximately 25% of month

EFFECTIVENESS OF CONTRACEPTIVE METHODS

Sterilization, Implant, IUD
Injection, Pill, Ring, Patch
Diaphragm, Condoms, Sponge, Cervical cap
Spermicides, Fertility awareness, Withdrawal

ectopic pregnancy

Any concepts that implants and grows outside the uterine cavity

SYMPTOMS:
1. Amenorrhea
2. Abnormal uterine bleeding spotting (may be dark brown to tarry)
3. Abdominal/pelvic complaints
4. Unilateral lower quadrant pain
5. Lower back pain or shoulder pain
6. Hemodynamic changes in vital signs (shock-rupture)

PHYSICAL EXAMINATION:
- Tender adnexa with possible palpable mass
- Positive cervical motion tenderness
- Uterine enlargement
- Positive peritoneal signs if rupture has occured and, perhaps, vaginal bleeding

DIANOSTIC TESTS:
- Serum hCG (quantitative)
- CBC, type, and RhUltrasound
- Other preoperative labs

TREATMENT:
Refer

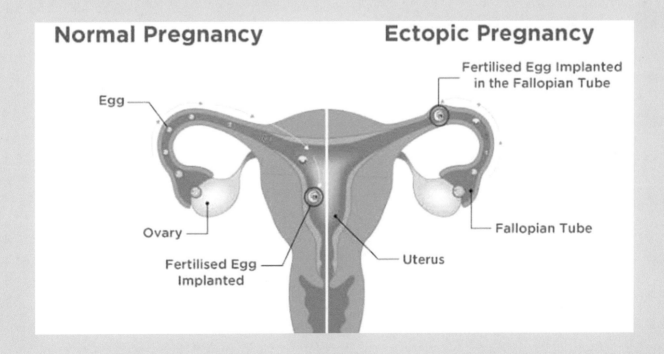

Normal Pregnancy

Egg

Ovary

Fertilised Egg Implanted

Ectopic Pregnancy

Fertilised Egg Implanted in the Fallopian Tube

Fallopian Tube

Uterus

Intrauterine pregnancy

40-week process by which an embryo grows and develops into an infant within the uterus of the mother

SYMPTOMS:
 1. *FIRST TRIMESTER (TO 12 WEEKS)*
 * Amenorrhea
 * Nausea
 * Vomiting
 * Fatigue
 * Breast tenderness
 * Urinary frequency
 2. *SECOND TRIMESTER (13 TO 27 WEEKS)*
 * Fetal movement
 * Abdominal discomfort
 * Change in skin pigmentation (*Chloasma*)
 * Syncopal episodes
 3. *THIRD TRIMESTER (28 TO 40 WEEKS)*
 * Abdominal growth
 * Braxton-Hicks contractions
 * Urinary frequency with descent of presenting part
 * Increased respiratory effort until descent

PHYSICAL EXAMINATION:
 1. *FIRST TRIMESTER:*
 * Softening of cervix (Goodell's sign)
 * Cervical cyanosis (Chadwick's sign)
 * Softening of cervicouterine junction (Hegar's sign)
 * Breast enlargement
 * Fetal heart tones (FHT) by 10 to 12 weeks
 2. *SECOND TRIMESTER:*
 * Striae may appear on breasts, hips, or abdomen
 * Fundus palpable at umbilicus at 20 weeks gestation and grows approximately 1 cm per week thereafter
 * Leopold maneuvers possible after 20 weeks
 3. *THIRD TRIMESTER:*
 * Lightening may occur up to three to four weeks prior to labor
 * Loss of mucus plug/bloody show prior to labor by approximately 1 week
 * May experience increase in Braxton-Hick contractions/rupture of membranes

DIAGNOSTIC TESTS:
 1. Urine or serum pregnancy tests to confirm pregnancy
 2. Quantitative titers performed on serum hCG only
 3. Ultrasound
 4. First trimester and/or new visit
 * U/A
 * Urine C and S
 * CBC
 * Blood group and Rh
 * Antibody screening
 * Rubella (vaccine not to be given during pregnancy)
 * HbsAg
 * Syphilis testing screens
 * HIV
 * Specialty screening
 * PAP
 * Cervical cultures (STD screening, dating ultrasound for unsure dates and/or size unequal to dates, chrionic villus sampling CVS)

2. Second trimester: amniocentesis at 15 to 20 weeks if family history of chomosomal abnormalities or advanced maternal age

- Triple or quad screen (multiple marker test) at 16-20 weeks
- Triple screen: hCG, estriol, and alpha-fetoprotein
- Quad screen: hCG, estriol, alpha-fetoprotein, and inhibin-A
- Ultrasound for fetal survey at 18-20 weeks
- 1 hour GTT (or other glucose check) at 20 weeks if family history of diabetes or patient weight greater than 200 pounds

3. Third trimester: 1 hour GTT at 28 weeks for routine screening

- RhoGAM for un-sensitized Rh-negative mothers at 28 weeks
- Hemoglobin/hematocrti at 28-36 weeks dependent upon previous levels
- Nonstress tests (NST)/biphysical proile (BPP) as needed for assesment of fetal well-being
- Hepatitis B vaccine and group B strep test for each pregnancy

TREATMENT:

1. Scheduling of prenatal visits:
   - 0 to 28 weeks: every 4 weeks
   - 28 to 36 weeks: every 2 weeks
   - 36 weeks to delivery: every weeks
2. New OB visit:
   - Naegele's rule: 1 year-3 months + 7 days from last normal menstrual period
3. Return OB visits:
   - Labs: routine, plus urine for protein, glucose, and ketones at each visit

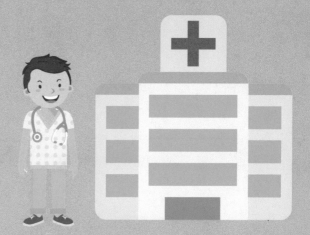

HIGH RISK REQUIRING CONSULTATION:

1. Pregnancy losses
2. Family history of genetic anomalies
3. Rh sensitization
4. Hemoglobinopathies
5. Thrombocytipenia
6. Multiple gestation
7. HIV
8. Uterine bleeding
9. Premature rupture of membranes
10. Pre-eclampis/PIH
11. Gestational diabetes/insulin dependent diabetes
12. Fetal presentation other tha vertex after 32-34 weeks
13. Intrauterine growth retardation
14. Previous preterm labor

PLACENTIA
Previa

Mal-implantation of the placenta in the lower uterine segment

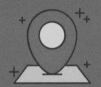 Bleeding usually occurs in the late second to early third trimester and often is precipitated by vaginal intercourse

SYMPTOMS:
1. Bleeding is painless
2. May occur immediately following vaginal intercourse
3. May have no precipitating factor
4. No evidence of contractions
5. No uterine tenderness
6. Often little to no fetal compromise unless bleeding is severe or other cause of distress

TESTS:
- Ultrasound for localization of placental implantation
- EFM to exclude fetal distress
- If bleeding is continous or severe, obtain CBC

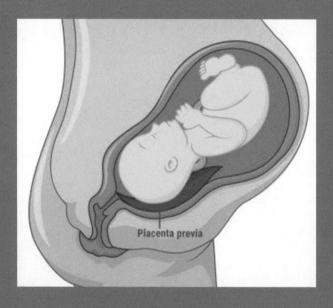

Placenta previa

TREATMENT:
- No bimanual exam: speculum examination only to determine extent of bleeding
- Hospitalization usually required
- NST/BPP while in hospital and the weekly
- Vaginal rest: NOTHING in the vagina
- If fetus is mature, anticipate delivery

Postpartum Complications

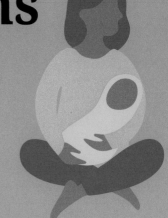

1. Pulmonary embolism (shortness of breath)
2. Postpartum hemorrhage
3. Postpartum depression
4. Mastitis (painful of the breast, usually due to staphylococcal species)

a) Symptomatic treatment (e.g., NSAID's, ice packs), antibiotic therapy (e.g., dicloxacillin, cephalexin, clindamycin)

Premature Labor

The occurrence of contractions after 20 weeks but before 37 weeks gestation wich result in the dilatation and/or effacement of the cervical os, contractions may or may not be perceived by the mother as painful or even present

RISK FACTORS:
- History of preterm delivery
- Genital and/or urinary tract infections
- Multiple gestation
- Poor weight gain, poor nutrition
- Drug use, especially cocaine and smoking
- Uterine structural abnormalities
- Cervical trauma
- Adolescent or advanced maternal AGE

SYMPTOMS:
- Uterine cramping that is intermittent or consistant
- Lower back pain
- Uterine contractions with a frequency or 10-12 minutes (5/hr)
- May experience vaginal spotting or change in vaginal discharge
- Cervical effacement/shortening and/ir dilatation

PREVENTION:
1. Reassessment of risk factors each trimester
2. Education regarding warning signs of premature labor

TREATMENT:
- Hospitalization if unable to stop contractions prior to cervical change
- Tocolytic therapy if cervical change occurs
- If less than 34 weeks and succesfully tocolysed, give B-methasone (steroid) injections twice a week to enhance fetal lung maturity, until 34 weeks
- Bed rest
- Vaginal rest and bed rest at home
- Weekly cervical checks

Pulmonary

DISORDERS

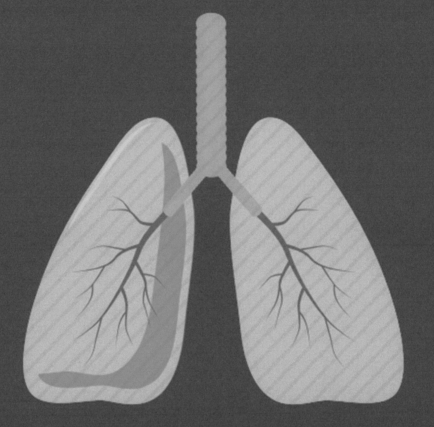

Acute bronchitis
Asthma
COPD
Cough etiologies and treatment
Cystic fibrosis
Pertussia
Pneumonia

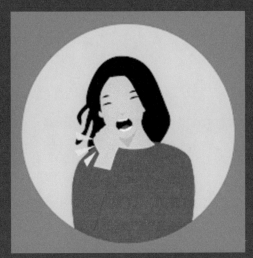

Acute BRONCHITIS

Inflammation of the bronchioles, bronchi, and trachea; usually follows an upper respiratory infection

SYMPTOMS

Cough due to acute inflammation of the trachea and large airways without evidence of pneumonia
Mildly ill-appearing
Lung auscultation may reveal wheezes, as well as rhonchi that typically improve with coughing
Fever

DIAGNOSTIC STUDIES

-Laboratory testing (usually not indicated in the evaluation of acute bronchitis)
-Leukocytosis is present in about 20% of patients.
-Chest X-Ray PA/Lateral is primarily used to rule out pneumonia.

INDICATIONS FOR CHEST RADIOGRAPHY IN ADULT PATIENTS WITH SYMPTOMS OF ACUTE BRONCHITIS

Dyspnea, bloody sputum, or rusty sputum color
Pulse > 100 beats per minute
Respiratory rate > 24 breaths per minute
Oral body temperature > 100°F (37.8°C)
Focal consolidation, egophony, or fremitus on chest examination

TREATMENT

-Antitussive such as dextromethorphan, guaifenesin, or honey and NSAIDs
-Antitussives have minimal benefit
-Beta agonists have minimal benefit
-Antibiotics are commonly prescribed, but usually not necessary

RECOMMENDATIONS

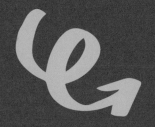

Use delayed prescription strategies, such as asking patients to call for or pick up an antibiotic or to hold an antibiotic prescription for a set amount of time
Address patient concerns in a compassionate manner
Discuss the expected course of illness and cough duration (two to three weeks)
Explain that antibiotics do not significantly shorten illness duration and are associated with adverse effects and antibiotic resistance
Discuss the treatment plan, including the use of non antibiotic medications to control symptoms
Describe the infection as a viral illness or chest cold

asthma

1st line treatment
- SABA: Albuterol or Levalbuterol (Xopenex) PRN

2nd line treatment
- Low-dose ICS
- Inhaled Corticosteroids: Fluticasone (Flovent) Mometasone (Asmanex) Budesonide (Pulmicort) Beclomethasone (Qvar

3rd line treatment
- Low-dose ICS plus LABA or Medium-dose ICS
- Inhaled Corticosteroids: Fluticasone (Flovent) Mometasone (Asmanex) Budesonide Pulmicort) Beclomethasone (Qvar)
- LABA: salmeterol, advair, symbicort, dulera, breo ellipta, serevent

4th line treatment
- Medium dose ICS plus LABA
- Inhaled Corticosteroids: Fluticasone (Flovent) Mometasone (Asmanex) Budesonide (Pulmicort) Beclomethasone (Qvar)
- LABA: salmeterol, advair, symbicort, dulera, breo ellipta, serevent

EXACERBATIONS

Can be classified as mild, moderate, severe, or life threatening.

5th line treatment
- Consider omalizumab for patients who have allergies
- Inhaled Corticosteroids: Fluticasone (Flovent) Mometasone (Asmanex) Budesonide)Pulmicort) Beclomethasone (Qvar)
- LABA: salmeterol, advair, symbicort, dulera, breo ellipta, serevent

6th line treatment
- High dose ICS plus LABA plus oral corticosteroid
- Consider Omalizumab for patients who have allergies

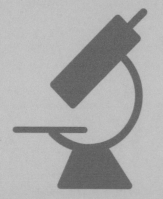

DIAGNOSTIC STUDIES

- Spirometer testing at least every 2 years
- Evidence of variable expiratory airflow limitation (reduced FEV1/FVC ratio)

COPD

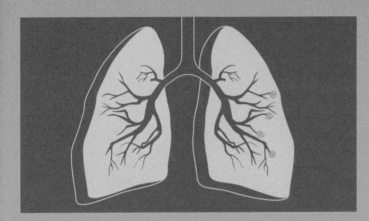

SIGNS & SYMPTOMS
Dyspnea
Chronic cough
Chronic sputum production
Recurrent lower respiratory tract infections

DIAGNOSTIC STUDIES

- Spirometer shows post bronchodilator (FEV1/FVC ratio <.70) Confirms diagnosis
-Chest -ray. PA/Lateral

1st Line Treatment
·Short-acting anticholinergic PRN or SABA PRN
·Short-acting anticholinergic: Combivent, anoro, spirivia, tudorza, lpratropium (Atrovent) 17 mcg 2 puffs inhaled qid max 12 puffs/day
·SABA: Albuterol / Levalbuterol

2nd Line Treatment
·Long-actin anticholinergic or LABA; plus rescuer inhaler
·LABA: salmeterol, advair, symbicort, dulera, breo ellipta, serevent
·Long-acting anticholinergic
·Aclidinium (Tudorza Pressair)
·Umeclidinium (Incruse Ellipta)
·Glycopyrrolate (Seebri Neohaler)

3rd Line Treatment
·ICS + LABA or LA anticholinergic; plus rescuer inhaler
·Inhaled corticosteroids: budesonide, mometasone, fluticasone
·LABA: salmeterol, advair, symbicort, dulera, breo ellipta, serevent
·Long-acting anticholinergic
·Aclidinium (Tudorza Pressair)
·Umeclidinium (Incruse Ellipta)
·Glycopyrrolate (Seebri Neohaler)

4th Line Treatment
·Inhaled Corticosteroids + LABA and/or LA anticholinergic; plus rescuer inhaler
·ICS + LABA or LA anticholinergic; plus rescuer inhaler
·Inhaled corticosteroids: budesonide, mometasone, fluticasone
·LABA: salmeterol, advair, symbicort, dulera, breo ellipta, serevent
·Long-acting anticholinergic
·Aclidinium (Tudorza Pressair)
·Umeclidinium (Incruse Ellipta)
·Glycopyrrolate (Seebri Neohaler)

EXACERBATIONS

Management of Exacerbations
CBC, sputum culture?
Bronchodilator/anticholinergic or both: nebulized?
Systemic corticosteroids (shorten recovery time, improve lung function)
Antibiotics for increased dyspnea, sputum production, purulence

Oral Steroids
CHRONIC use should be avoided!!!Unfavorable risk-to- benefit ratio

COUGH ETIOLOGIES AND TREATMENT

Cough Differential	
Acute (<3 weeks)	Chronic (>8 weeks)
Acute respiratory infection (bronchitis, sinusitis, PND)	Asthma: 2nd most common cause
Exacerbation of COPD, asthma	GERD: 1st, 2nd, or 3rd most common (depends on who you read)
Pneumonia	Infection: Pertussis, atypical pneumonia, TB
Pulmonary embolism	ACE inhibitors: dry cough 1-3 weeks after starting
Others	-Chronic bronchitis (almost always smokers) -Bronchiectasis (chronic cough, viscid sputum, bronchial wall thickening on CT scan) -Lung cancer: <2% of cases

Patients who warrant chest X-ray when acute cough is present

-Abnormal vital signs (increased RR or HR, temp >38°C, 100.4°F)
-Rales, consolidation -≥75 years of age with cough

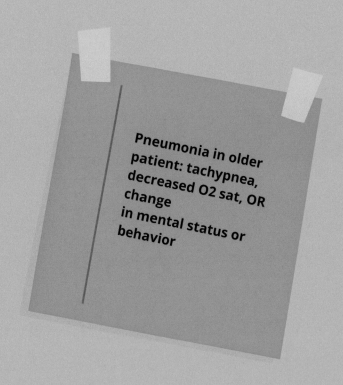

CYSTIC FIBROSIS

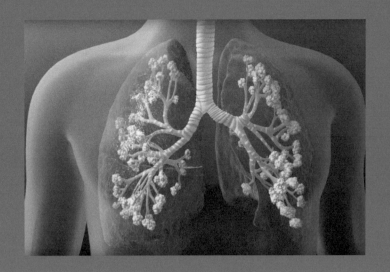

SIGNS AND SYMPTOMS

Viscid meconium (or meconium ileus) in new born.
Recurrent respiratory infection.
Large, liquid, bulky, foul stool (steatorrhea).
Salt-tasting skin
Chronic cough, rhinorrhea.
Hepatosplenomegaly.
Fat-soluble vitamin deficiencies.
Failure to thrive.
Delayed puberty.
Infertility.

DIAGNOSTIC STUDIES

-Pilocarpine iontophoresis sweat test.
-Pulmonary function tests (PFTSs): Obstructive pattern.
-Hyponatremic, hypochloremic dehydration (alkalosis).
-Chest radiograph: cystic lesions, atelectasis.

MANAGMENT

Referral for specially management

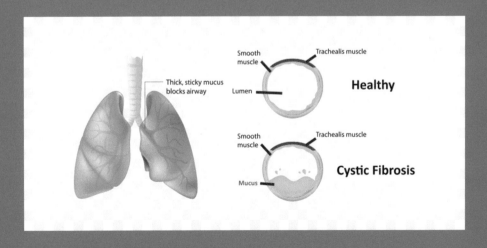

PERTUSSIA

SIGNS & SYMPTOMS

Whooping cough
Highly contagious
Uncontrollable and violent coughing which often makes
it hard to breathe
Cough persisting for more than two weeks
Paroxysmal cough
Post-tussive emesis
Recent pertussis exposure

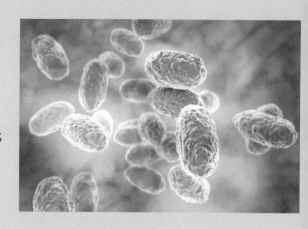

DIAGNOSTIC STUDIES

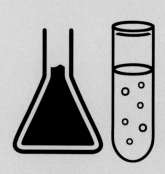

-First 2 weeks of cough order culture of nasal B. Pertussis
-0 to 3 weeks following cough onset order Test with PCR from NP
specimens
-2 to 8 weeks following cough onset order serology test.

TREATMENT

Azithromycin
Clarithromycin
Erythromycin
Trimethoprim-sulfamethoxasole

RECOMMENDATIONS

-CDC recommends pertussis
vaccines for infants, children, adolescents, and
adults. Give five doses of DTaP to children 2
months through 6 years of age.
-CDC recommends one dose of Tdap for those 11
years or older, with a preferred administration at
11 or 12 years of age.
-CDC also recommends Tdap for pregnant women
during each pregnancy, with a preferred
administration during the early part of gestational
weeks 27 through 36.

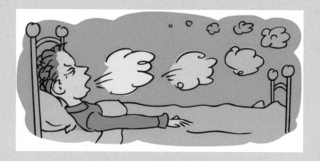

PNEUMONIA

PNEUMONIA PNEUMONIA PNEUMONIA PNEUMONIA PNEUMONIA

SIGNS & SYMPTOMS

Tachypnea, tachycardia, dyspnea, lung findings suggestive of pneumonia

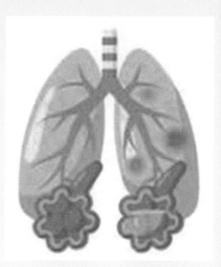

DIAGNOSTIC STUDIES

-X-Ray not necessary if responding appropriately to treatment
-Consider X-Ray follow-up in 7-12 weeks after treatment if: >40 years, in smokers to confirm resolution and exclude underlying diseases, malignancy

TREATMENT

-Minimally 5 days --- when afebrile for 48-72 h and clinically stable
-Treatment is about 5-10 days •
·   When should symptoms resolve?
Clinical symptoms: fever usually resolves by Day 3; cough, fatigue may persist -14 days depending on patient
-Re-evaluate after 48-72 hours
if poor response to treatment

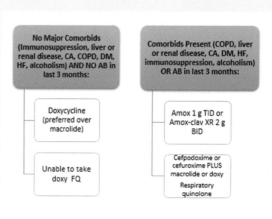

COMMON ANTIBIOTICS FOR CAP

Antibiotic Class	Generic Names	Examples
Respiratory Fluoroquinolones "floxacin"	Moxifloxacin Gemifloxacin Levofloxacin	Avelox Factive Levaquin
Macrolides "mycin"	Azithromycin Clarithromycin	Zithromax Biaxin
Tetracycline's	Doxycycline	Monodox
Beta Lactams	Amoxicillin Amox with clavulanate	Amoxil Augmentin

RECOMMENDATIONS

-PPSV 23 only: Adults 19-64 years at increased risk of pneumococcal disease (asthma,
-COPD, smokers, CV dx (not HTN), DM, liver disease, etc.)
-PCV13, then PPSV 23 in 1 year: Adults ≥65
-PCV 13, then PPSV 23 in 8 weeks, then PPSV 23 in 5 years: Adults 19-64 with asplenia, immunocompromising conditions, CSF leaks, cochlear implants

Respiratory Disorders

Respiratory Disorders

Common cold
Influenza "flu"
Mononucleosis
Nose bleeds
Pharyngitis/Tonsillitis
Sinusitis (Rhinosinusitis)

COMMON COLD

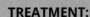

SIGNS AND SYMPTOMS:

1. Rhinorrhea
2. Sneezing
3. Nasal and sinus blockage
4. Headache
5. Sore throat
6. Cough

TREATMENT:
- Supportive care
- Hydration, steam/humidifier
- Fever and pain: Tylenol, Motrin, Advil
- Warm salt water gargles

INFLUENZA (''FLU'')

Acute, febrile illness caused by infection with influenza type A and B virus

SIGN AND SYMPTOMS

Fever
Headache
Myalgia
Coryza
Anorexia
Malaise
Cough

LABORATORY DIAGNOSTICS

Nasal or throat swab or sputum specimens

TREATMENT
- Supportive care: Antipyretics
- Oseltamivir (Tamiflu oral)
- Zanamivir (Relenza inhlaler) not recommended in patients with underlying
  respiratory disease (asthma, COPD) due to the risk of bronchospasm

MONONUCLEOSIS

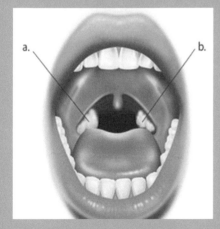

SIGN AND SYMPTOMS

1. Fever
2. Chilis
3. Malaise/fatigue
4. Anorexia
5. Pharyngitis (most severe symptom)
6. White tonsillar exudates
7. Adenopathy/lymphadenopathy (posterior cervical region)
8. Splenomegaly (usually during the 2nd week of illness)

TREATMENT:
- Supportive care
- Prednisone/ steroid taper for severely enlarged tonsils
- Contact sports avoided (3 weeks to months) splenic rupture may occur

LABORATORY DIAGNOSTICS:
- Monospot positive
- Increased WBC with relative lymphocytosis and neutropenia

nose bleeds (epistaxis)

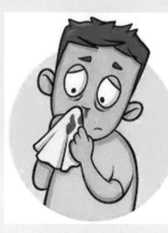

SIGNS AND SYMPTOMS:
-Bleeding from only one nostril
-Signs of excessive blood loss
-Dizziness
-Weakness
-Confusion
-Fainting

TREATMENT
Sit upright
Constant pressure to the nose
Apply ice

pharyngintis/tonsillitis

SYMPTOMS:
-Erythematous pharynx
-Rhinorrhea
-Cough
-Anterior cervical adenopathy
-Fever
-Painful throat
-Macropapular rash

DIAGNOSTIC STUDIES
-Rapid strep test
-Monospot
-CBC with differential

TREATMENT
1. Fluids/hydration
2. SALT WATER GARGLES
3. Aspirin/Tylenol
4. Antibiotics for streptococcal infection (Penicillin V, Erythromycin)
5. Ceftriaxone for genococcal infection
6. Refer

sinusitis (rhinosinusitis)

SYMPTOMS
Red nasal mucosa
Pain/pressure over face, nose, cheeks, teeth
Purulent nasal drainage
Fever
Tenderness over sinuses
Headache in supine or bending position
Foul-smelling nasal or post-nasal drainage

DIAGNOSTIC STUDIES
Culture as needed
Radiographs/CT
Decreased transillumination
TREATMENT
Hydration, oral decongestants/antihistamines
Analgesics
Antibiotics only for bacterial cases
Supportive care

SEXUALLY
TRANSMITTED INFECTIONS/DISEASES

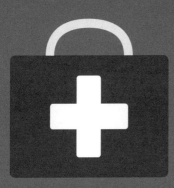

- <u>Acquired immune deficiency syndrome (AIDS)</u>
- <u>Chancroid</u>
- <u>Chlamydia</u>
- <u>Genital warts (condyloma acuminata)</u>
- <u>Gonorrhea</u>
- <u>Hepatitis B</u>
- <u>Herpes</u>
- <u>Lymphogranuloma venerum LGV</u>
- <u>Mollusium contagiosum</u>
- <u>Syphilis</u>

Acquired Immune Deficiency Syndrome (AIDS)

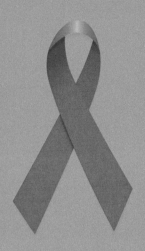

SYMPTOMS:

1. Flu-like symptoms: Think seroconversion (process of converting from HIV negative to HIV positive; the process takes approximately 3 weeks to 6 months)
2. Early s/s inculde: fever, night sweats, and weight loss
3. *It is more a constellation of signs/symptoms than any single one that is suspicious for AIDS= CD4 <200 cells/ml, and/or the presence of an opportunistic infection

LABORATORY/DIAGNOSTICS

1. ELISA for initial screening sensivity > 99.9%
2. Western Blot test is confirmatory
3. Latest recommended HIV tests:
4. - HIV-1/2 antigen/antibody combination immunoassay; if positive, proceed to:
5. -HIV-1/2 antibody differentiation immunoassay
6. 4. Absolute CD4 lymphocyte count: NORMAL> 800 cells/ml
7. 5. CD4lymphocyte percentage
8. -Risk of progression to AIDS high when <20%
9. 6. Viral load
10. -PCR: based quantitative copies of HIV-branched DNA or RNA
11. -Results correlate closely with progression of HIV
12. -Ideally should be "zero" or "undetectable"

TREATMENT:

1. Therapy for opportunistic infections
2. -Treat infection as it occurs
3. -Bactrim for pneumocystis jiroveci pneumonia prophylaxis
4. 2. Antiretroviral treatment
5. -Combination therapy is standard (Active Antiretroviral Therapy AART)
6. -When to start AART remains somewhat controversial CDC and DHHS recommend starting medications at the time of HIV+diagnosis
7. 3. Monitor for the danger of drug resistance: must be taken exactly as prescribed

chancroid

SYMPTOMS

1. WOMEN: Usually asymptomatic
2. MEN: Single (or multiple) superficial, painful ulcer, surrounded by an erythematous halo
3. Ulcers may be necrotic or severly erosive

DIAGNOSIS

Painful genital ulcers by inspection or culture

TREATMENT

1. Azithromycin (Zithromax) 1 gram by mouth x 1 dose
2. Ceftriaxone (Rocephin) 250 mg IM x 1 dose
3. Ciprofloxacin (Cipro) 500 mg by mouth twice a day x 3 days

chlamydia

A parasitic STD caused by Chlamydia trachomatis that produces serious reproductive tract complications

SYMPTOMS

FEMALES:
- Dysuria
- intramenstrual spotting
- Postcoital bleeding
- Dyspareunia: painful intercourse
- Vaginal discharge

MALES:
- Dysuria
- Thick, cloudy penile discharge
- Resticular pain

DIAGNOSIS

1. Chlamydia culture most the most definitive test (3 to 9 days for results)
2. Enzyme immunoassay (EIA) methods preferred (low cost, 30 to 120 min for results)

TREATMENT

1. Azithromycin (Zithromax) 1 gram by mouth x 1 dose
2. Doxycycine (Vibramycin) 100 mg by mouth twice a day x 7 days
3. Alternatives: erythromycin, ofloxacin, levofloxacin
4. Report to the health department

Genital Warts
(CONDYLOMA ACUMINATA)
Human papillomavirus (HPV)

SYMPTOMS

Single (or multiple) soft, fleshy, papillary, or sessile, painless keratinized growth around anus, vulvovaginal area, penis, urethra, or perineum

DIAGNOSIS

1. Clinical presentation, perhaps atypical squamous cell of undetermined significance (ACUS) or squamous intraepithelial lesion (SIL) on PAP smear
2. Colposcopy useful in diagnosing flat lesions
3. May need to biopsy if at risk for cervial intraepithelial neoplasia (CIN)

TREATMENT

1. Keratolytic agents: podophyllin (Pododerm), trinchloroacetic acid (TCA), or bichloracetic acid (BCA)
2. Referral for cryotherapy, laser therapy, electrocautery, or excision

PREVENTION

1. Gardasil (Human papillomavirus quadrivalent types 6, 11, 16 and 18 vaccination):
2. -Gardasil 9 is a 9-valent for prevention of cervical, vulvar, vaginal, and anal cancer
3. -Indicated for females and males ages 9 to 26 years
4. -Given in 3 injections
5. 2. Cervarix (Human papillomavirus bivalent types 16 and 18 vaccination):
6. -Indicated for females ages 10 to 25 years
7. -Same as above

GONORRHEA

INCIDENCE

Produces urethritis in men and cervicitis in women, leading cause of infertility among females

SYMPTOMS

FEMALES:
Dysuria, urinary frequency, mucopurulent vaginal discharge (green), labial pain and swelling, lower abdominal pain, fever, abnormal menstrua periods, and dysmenorrhea

MALES:
Dysuria, frequency, white/yellow-green penile discharge, and testicual pain

LABORATORY/ DIAGNOSTICS

1. Gram stain of discharge smear shows gram-negative diplococci and WBC
2. Cervical culture for N. gonorrhoeae using modified Thayer-Martin media

TREATMENT

1. Ceftriaxone (Rocephin) 250 mg IM x 1 dose to ttreat gonorrhea
2. Azithromycin (Zithromax) 1 gram orally x 1 dose to cover chlamydia
3. Report to the health department

HEPATITIS B

PREVENTION

Three commercially available hepatitis B preventive vaccines:
- Heplisav-B: 2 doses, at least 4 weeks apart
-Recombiax HB: 3 doses at 0, 1, and 6 months
-Engerix-B: 3 doses, at 0, 1, and 2 months

TREATMENT

1. Supportve and symptomatic care
2. Hepatitis B immune globulin (HBIG) 0.06 ml/kg IM in single dose within 14 days of exposure (earlier administration may be more effective)

HERPES

CAUSES:
1. Herpes simplex virus type 1: associated with infection of lips, face, and mucosa
2. Herpes simplex virus type 2: associated with the negitalia
3. Transmission: direct contact with active lesions or virus-containing fluid (salive or cervical secretions)

SYMPTOMS:
1. Initial: fever, malaise, dysuria, painful/pruritic ulcers for usually 12 days
2. Recurrent: less painful/prurtic ulcers for usually 5 days
3. Herpetic whitlow: HSV-1 =60%, HSV-2 =40%

DIAGNOSTICS:
1. Papanicolaou or tzanck stain
2. Viral culture is most defenitive

TREATMENT:
-Symptomatic treatment with drying and antipruritic agents
-Acyclovir (Zovirax) recommended for topical, oral, and IV use
-Famciclovir
-Valacyclovir: especially useful for asymptomatic viral shedding of HSV2

LYMPPHOGRANULOMA VENEREUM

CAUSE:
Immunotypes L1, L2, L3 of chlamydia trachomatis

SYMPTOMS:
2 to 3 mm painless vesicle, bubo, or non-indurated ulcer
Regional adenopathy follows in approximately 1 month and is the most common finding
Stiffness and aching in groin followed by unilateral swelling of inguinal region

DIAGNOSIS:
May be confused with chancroid
Definitive diagnosis requires isolatin C, trachomatis from an appropiate specimen

TREATMENT:
Doxycycline (Vibramycin) 100 mg orally twice a day x 21 days
Aspirate buboes to prevent ulcerations

molluscum contagiosum

SYMPTOMS:
1. Lesions are 1 to 5 mm, smooth, rounded, firm, shiny flesh-colored to pearly-white papules
2. Commonly seen on trunk and anogenital region

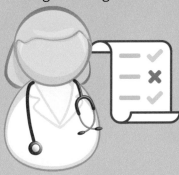

DIAGNOSIS:
Inspection and microscopic exam

TREATMENT:
Cryoanesthesia with liquid nitrogen: most popular method, may resolve without scarring

syphilis

SEROLOGIC TESTS:
1. Nonrtreponemal: VDRL/RPR
2. Treponemal:
3. - Fluorescent treponemal antibody absorption (FTA-ABS)
4. -Microhemagglutination assay for antibody to T. pallidum (MHA-TP)

TREATMENT:
1. Primary, secondary, or early syphilis of less than 1 year duration: benzathine penicillin G 2.4 million units IM
2. Late, latent , and indeterminate lenght: tertiary stage: benzathine penicillin G 2.4 million units IM weekly x 3 weeks
3. Penicillin allergic: doxycycline 100 mg orally twice a day or erythromycin 500 mg orally four times a day
4. Report to the health department

FOUR CLINICAL STAGES OF SYPHILIS:
1. *Primary*
2. - Chancre is painless
3. -Indurated ulcer
4. -Located at the site of exposure
5. *2. Secondary*
6. -Flu-like symptoms
7. -Highly variable skin rash
8. -Malaise, anorexia, alopecia, arthralgias
9. *3. Latent: seropositive, but asymptomatic*
10. *4. Tertiary:*
11. -Leukoplakia
12. -Cardiac insuffiency
13. -Aortic aneurysm
14. -Meningitis, hemiparesis, hemiplegia

Skin disorders

Acne
Bacterial infections
Herpes zoster (shingles)
Keratosis and skin cancers
Scabies
Other

ACNE

TREATMENT:
Non-pharmacologic therapies
-Wash several times daily with mild soap

Pharmacologic therapies
-Benzoyl peroxide
-Azelaic acid
-Tretinoin

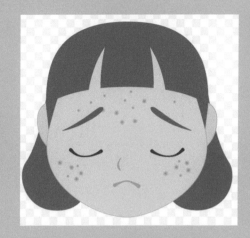

BACTERIAL INFECTIONS

FOLLICULITIS
Inflammation of the hair follicle

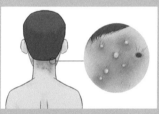

CELLULITIS
Dicloxacilin or cephalexin
Clindamycin or a macrolide for patients allergic to penicillin

HIDRADENITIS SUPPURATIVA
Staph aureus infection commonly in the groin or axilla

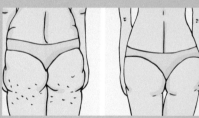

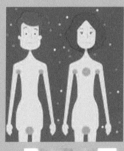

IMPETIGO
Honey-colored crusts at the edge

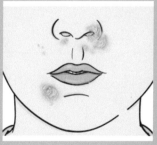

ERYSIPELAS
Usually caused by streptococcus

PARONYCHIA
Staphylococci around the nail fold

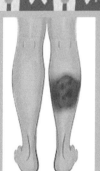

FURUNCLE
Staphylococcus aureus

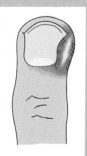

SYMPTOMS
Regional lymphadenopathy
Swelling
Rednes
Pustules
Pain
Warmth
Vesicles
Purulent drainage

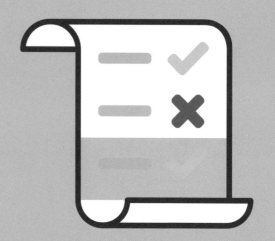

DIAGNOSTIC STUDIES
Culture if necessary

TREATMENT
Incision and drainage, as warranted
First generation cephalosporin
Penicillinase-resistant penicillin
Alternatives: Clindamycin or
amoxicillin-clavulate

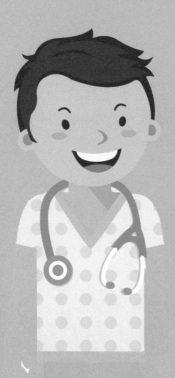

Herpes Zoster (Shingles)

SIGNS AND SYMPTOMS:
Regional lymphadenopathy may be present

TREATMENT:
-Acyclovir
-Famciclovir
-Valacyclovir
-Ocular involvement, immediate referral to ophtahalmologist
-Post-herpic neuralgia: gabapentin (naurontin) pregablin (lyrica)
-Shingrix: indicated for all adults > 50 years of age, regardless of previous shingles or Zotavax vaccine, 2 dose regimen with 2nd dose given 2 to 6 months after the initial dose

Keratosis and Skin Cancers

Basal cell carcinoma:
Shave/punch biopsy and surgical excision

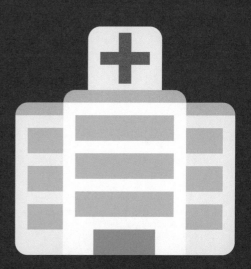

Squamous cell carcinoma: *Biopsy and surgical excision (Mohs)*

Malignant melanoma:
biopsy and surgical excision

SCABIES

INFECTION OF HUMAN SKIN BY MITES, USUALLY SARCOPATES SCABIEI

INITIAL TREATMENT

-Topical Permethrin

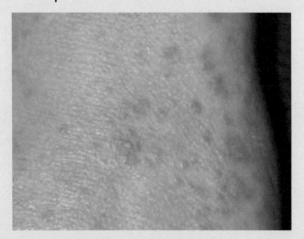

ASSESSMENT FINDINGS

-Itching (more noticeable at nighttime)
-Small itching blisters in a thin line
-Mite burrows between finger webbing, feet, wrists, axilla, scrotum, penis, waist, and/or buttocks

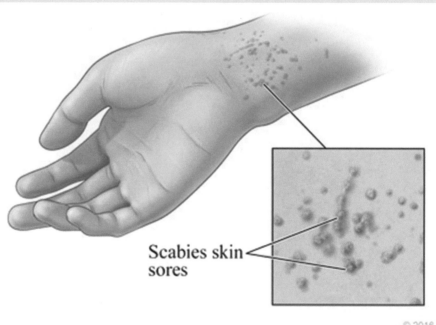

Scabies skin sores

Other common skin disorders

Eczema (Atopic Dermatitis)

Chronic skin doncition characterized by intense pruritus
TREATMENT:
Topical steroids, rubbed in well (clobetasol cream/lotion)

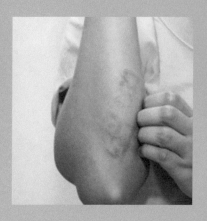

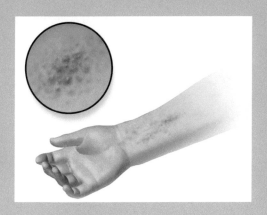

Allergic Contact Dermatitis

Acute of chronic condition characterized by inflammation at the site of contact with chemical allergens
TREATMENT:
Topical steroids
Do not scrub with soap and water
Prednisone taper if severe

Psoriasis

Benign yhyperproliferative inflammation of the skin that can be acute or chronic
Itching, red, precisely defined plaques with silvery scales
TREATMENT:
Topical for scalp
Topical steroids
UVB light exposure

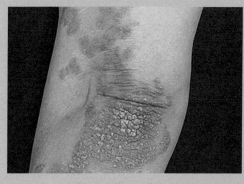

Pityriasis Rosea

Pruritc rash found on trunk and proximal extremities
Lesions follow a Christmas tree pattern
TREATMENT
Oral antihistamines
Topical antipruritic
Cool compress
Topical steroids
UVB light
Oral erythromycin

Warts

Benigns apidermal neoplasms caused by human papillomavirus (HPV)
Transmitted by direct contact
TREATMENT
Salicylic acid
Liquid nitrogen
Electrocautery
Tretinoin cream
Refer to dermatologist

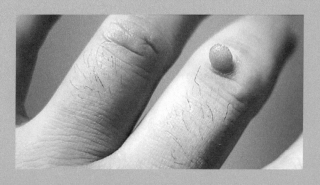

Tinea Capitis

Selenium 2.5% shampoo
Oral terbinafine, itraconazole or fluconazole
Griseofulvin

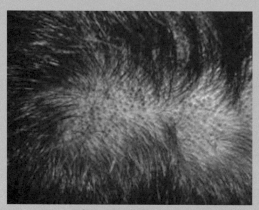

Tinea Corporis (ringworm)

Topical antifungals

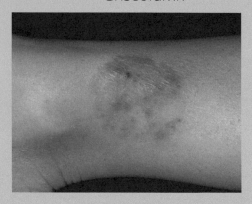

Tinea Cruris

Topical antifungals
Oral antifungals for severe cases

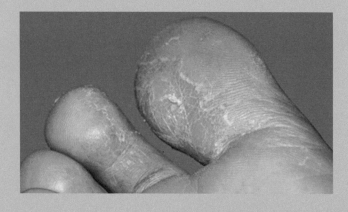

Tinea Pedis

Miconazole or clotrimazole

Tinea Unguium

Oral antifungals

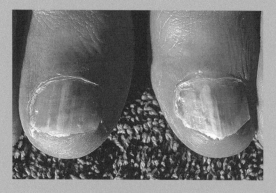

Tinea Versicolor

Topical selenium sulfide
Topical antifungals

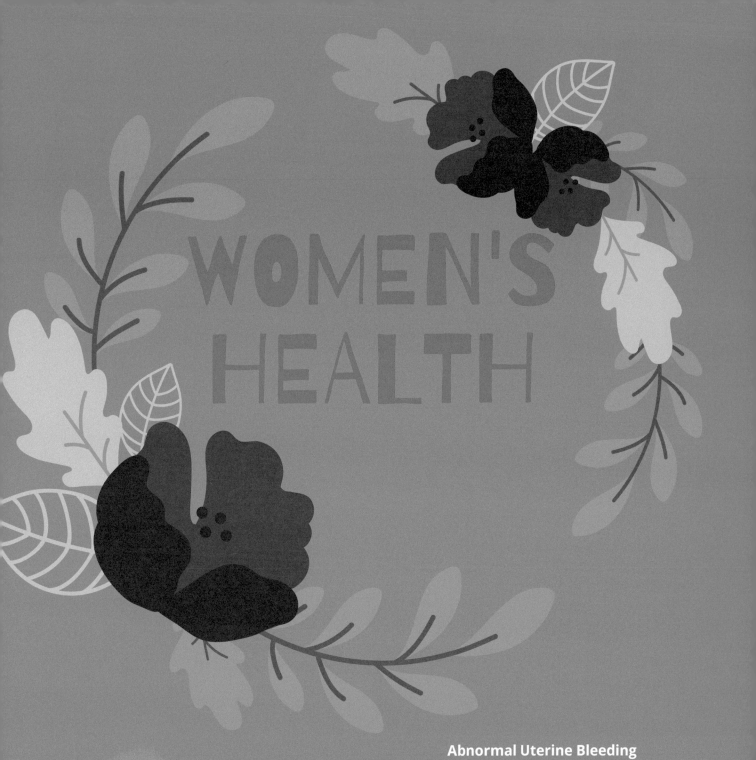

WOMEN'S HEALTH

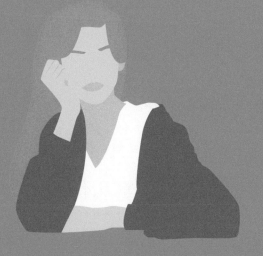

Abnormal Uterine Bleeding
Amenorrhea
Breast Cancer
Breast Cancer Screening
Cervical Cancer Screening for Average/Risk Woman
Dysmenorrhea
Fibrocystic Breast Disease
Menopause
Pelvic Inflammatory (PID)
Polycystic Ovarian Syndrome (PCOS)
Premenstrual Syndrome (PMS)/ Premenstrual Dysphoric
Disorder (PDD)
Systemic Lupus Erythematosus (SLE)
Vulvovaginitis

ABNORMAL UTERINE BLEEDING

Heavy bleeding may also be result of other problems such as polycystic ovarian disease, immature hypothalamic-pituitary-ovarian

PALM-COEIN (International Federation of Gynecology and Obstetrics (FIGO)

Polyps: Presence of endometrial-type glands and stroma within the myometrium
-Presentation: Intermenstrual and post-coital spotting
Adenomyosis: Endometrium breaks trhough the wall of the myometrium
-Presentation: Pain with periods and/or dyspareunia, chronic pelvic pain, heavy menstrual bleeding
Leiomyoma: Benign neoplasms of smooth muscle
-Presentation: Heavy menstrual bleeding
Malignancy and hyperplasia: Epithelial neoplasms of the endometrium
-Presentations: Any bleeding in postmenopausal women, any abnormal uterine bleeding age 45 to menopause, persistent abnormal uterine bleeding in those younger than 45 years of age

SYMPTOMS:
Evaluate for pregnancy
Evaluate for uterine bleeding

Coagulopathy: Spectrum of possibilities ancluiding deficient or defective clotting factors, platelets
Ovulatory dysfunction: Abnormal, irregular (with less than 9 menses/year)
-Physiological
-Pathologic
Endometrial causes: Idiopathic or endometritis
Iatrogenic causes: Chronic steroid use, contraceptives, containing progestin, intrauterine contraception

DIAGNOSTIC STUDIES:
Initial hCG (quantitive)
Prolactin
Thyroid functions (TSH)
CBC
STD screening

TREATMENT:
Consult refer

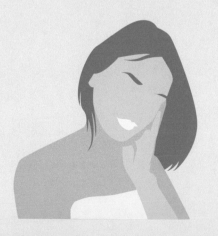

Amenorrhea

The absence of menstrual flow
PRIMARY: Abscence of menarche by age 16
SECONDARY: Cessation of menstrual flow after the establishment of normal menstrual cycling

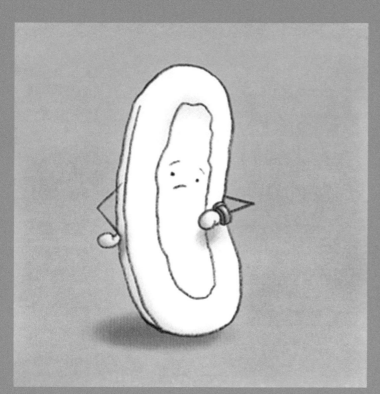

SYMPTOMS:
Primary: Abscence of menarche
Abscence of secondary sex characteristics
Abnormal growth & development

Secondary: Absence of expected menses with a history of regular cycles

DIAGNOSTIC TESTS:
Primary: Consider pregnancy test
Refer to endocrinologist

Secondary: Pregnancy test
Referral for other studies

Breast Cancer

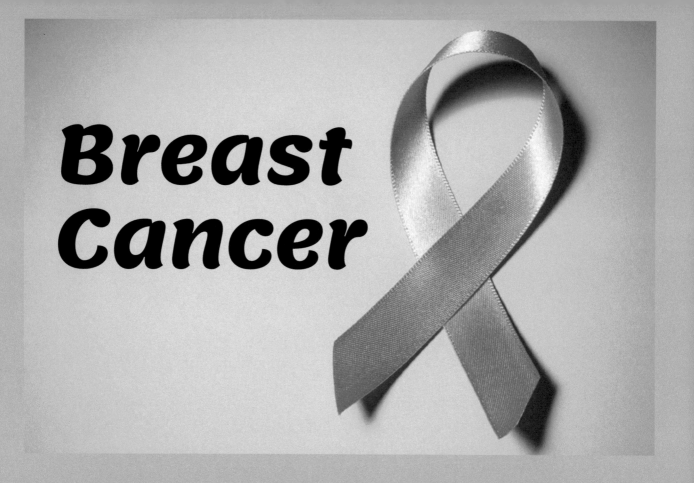

SYMPTOMS

1. Non-tender, painless mass
2. Asymptomatic, later symptoms include pain, erythema, dimpling, ulceration, nipple retraction

PHYSICAL EXAMINATION

- Non-tender with poorly defined borders
- May also find dimpling, nipple retractions, bloody discharge, hymphadenopathy
- May have bloody nipple discharge

DIAGNOSTIC TESTS

- Mamography
- FNA cytology

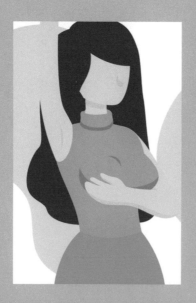

TREATMENT

Refer for:
- Surgery
- Chemotherapy
- Radiation
- Hormonal therapy

BREAST CANCER SCREENING
BREAST CANCER SCREENING

When to begin?	How often?	When to end?	Clinical breast exam?	Self-breast exam?
At ages 40 to 44	Annually for ages 45 to 54 Every 2 years after age 55	Continue as long as the woman is in good health and expected to live 10 more years or lnger	For ages 20 to 39 every 3 years. Annyally starting at age 40	Optional beginning at age 21. Women should be informed of potential benefits and harms

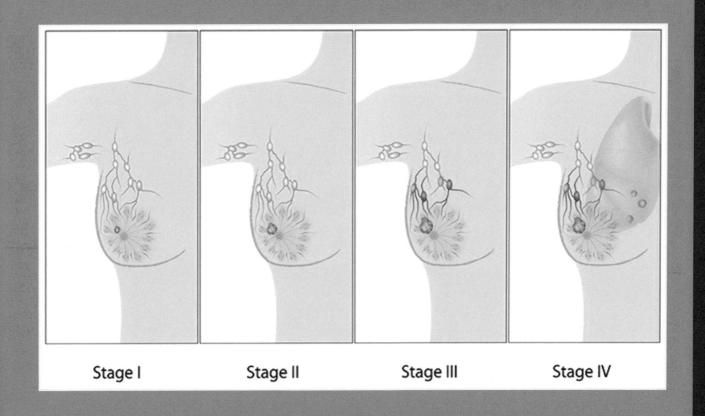

| Stage I | Stage II | Stage III | Stage IV |

FIBROCYSTIC BREAST DISEASE

Benign breast condition with increased growth and fibrosis of breast tissue

SYMPTOMS

Breast tenderness

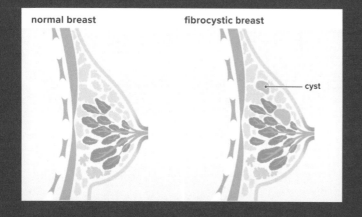

normal breast   fibrocystic breast

cyst

PHYSICAL EXAMINATION

-Tenderness to area
-Mobile
-May be round or nodular, soft or firm
-Nipple discharge usually clear

DIAGNOSTIC TESTS

-Mamography
-FNA cytology

TREATMENT

Warm soaks TID
Low sodium diet
Vitamin supplements
Hormonal therapy
Surgical intervention

MENOPAUSE

Cessation of ovarian function through biological aging, surgical removal, chemotherapy, and/or radiation

SYMPTOMS

- Skin: dryness, loss of elasticity, decreased sebaceous gland activity, changes in pigmentation
- CV: atherosclerosis, coronary artery disease
- Breast: decrease in tone, size
- Neuroendocrine: vasomotor symptoms (hot flashes, flushing, night swats), mood changes, depression, sleep disturbances
- Skeletal: osteoporosis

GENITOURINARY SYNDROME OF MENAPAUSE (GSM):
term used to describe changes to the vagina, vulva, and bladder
1) Genital dryness, burning, and irritation
2) Sexual complaints (dyspareunia and/or lack of lubrication)
3) Urinary symptoms (urgency, dysuria, and recurring UTI's)

TREATMENT

1) HORMONAL THERAPY (HT)/ MENOPAUSAL HOROMONE THERAPY (MHT)
-Estrogen therapy: for patients without a uterus due to a hysterectomy
-Estrogen plus progestogen therapy: progestogen is added to ET to protect women with a uterus against endometrial cancer from estrogen alone
-Encourage exercise, calcium supplementations, and healthy diet
2) CONTRAINDICATIONS FOR HT
-Breast cancer
-Endometrial cancer
-CAD/CHD (including dypertriglyceridemia)
-Venous thromboembolic disorders
-Active liver disease
-Unexplained vaginal bleeding
-Endometriosis and/or fibroids
3) NON-HORMONAL TREATMENT OF VASOMOTOR SYMPTOMS
-Paroxetine (7.5 mg/day) FDA approved

POLYCYSTIC OVARIAN SYNDROME (PCOS)

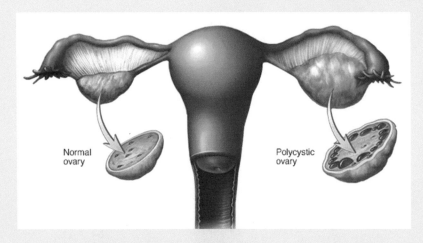

SYMPTOMS

1. Menstrual irregularity
2. Infertility
3. Hirsutism
4. Obesity and metabolic syndrome
5. Acne

ASSOCIATED CONDITIONS

1. DIabetes, metabolic syndrome
2. Heart and blood vessel complications
3. Uterine cancer
4. Sleep apnea

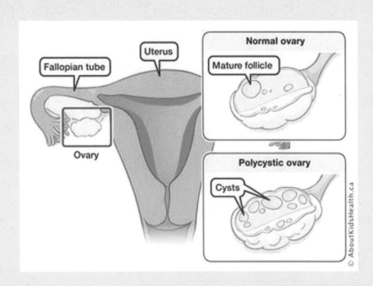

TREATMENT

Lifestyle changes
Pharmacologic interventions:
a) Oral contraceptives for menstrual regulation
b) Insulin-sensitizing medication
c) Hair removal treatment
d) Acne treatment

Systemic Lupus Erythematosus (SLE)

PERINGUAL ERYTHEMA

FINGERTIP LESIONS

ANOREXIA

ALOPECIA

FEVER

VASCULITIS

MALAISE

NEPHRITIS

JOINT SYMPTOMS OFTEN EARLY MANIFESTATION

OCULAR MANIFESTATION

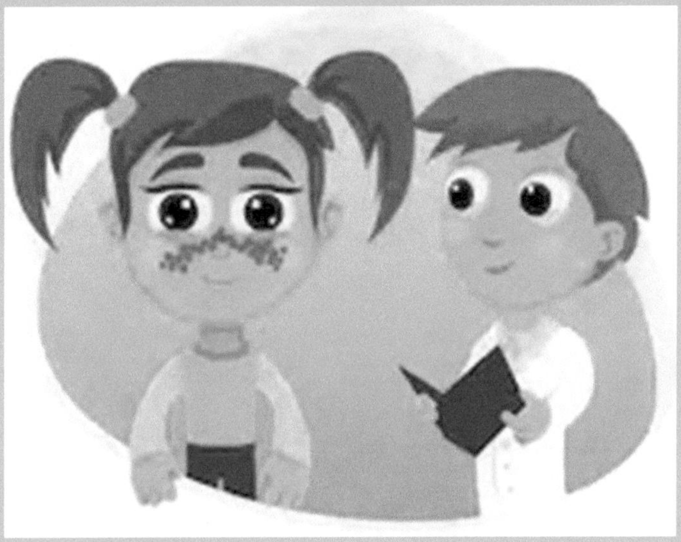

PERICARDIAL MANIFESTATION

WEIGHT LOSS

BUTTERFLY RASH

PULMONARY MANIFESTATION

ADBOMINAL PAINS, ILEUS, PERITONITIS

SPLINTER HEMORRHAGES

LABORATORY/ DIAGNOSTICS

ANA+in= 95% PATIENTS
Antiphospholipid antibodies
Anemia, leukopenia, and
thrombocytopenia are often
present

TREATMENT

- For mild symptoms: bed rest,
midafternoon naps, avoidance of fatigue
-Sun protection
-Topical glucocorticoid for isolated skin
lesions
-NSAIDS, hydroxychloroquine,
glucocorticoids and other therapies

Name:		Age:
Height:	Weight:	BMI:

Subjective
Historian:
Present Concerns/CC:

Child Profile
Sexual History:
ADL's:
Safety Practices:

HPI:

Medications:

PMH: None
Allergies:
Chronic Illnesses/Major Traumas:

Hospitalizations/Surgeries:

Family History:

Social History:

ROS

General

Cardiovascular

Skin

Respiratory

Eyes

Gastrointestinal

Ears

Genitourinary/Gynecological

Nose/Mouth/Throat

Musculoskeletal

Breast

Heart rate:_____ Blood Pressure:_____ Temperature_____

Respiration Rate:_____ Oxygen Saturation:_____%

Reason for Visit:_____

Neurological:

 Heme/Lymph/Endo

Psychiatric

Lab Tests

Diagnosis

Plan/Therapeutics

Patient Education

Vaccines/Medications

Follow Up

Medications

- Olmesartan 10-40mg QD
- Lisinopril 2.5-40mg QD
- Valsartan 80-320mg QD
- Losartan 25-100mg QD
- Metoprolol 25-200mg
- Carvedilol 3.125-80
- Propanolol 10-80mg
- Hydrochlorothiazide 12.5-50mg QD
- Hydralazine 10-100mg QID
- Amlodipine 2.5-10mg QD

- Atorvastatin QHS
- Rosuvastatin QHS
- Fenofibrate QHS
- Lovaza 2tabs/BID

- Ceterizine 10mg QD
- Montelukast 10mg QHS
- Flonase 2puff/BID
- Saline nasal spray PRN

- Symbicort 2puff/BID
- Albuterol Q4-6H PRN
- Pro-Air Q4-6H PRN

- Omnicef (cefdinir) 300mg Q12H ✳
- Augmentin 875/125mg Q12H ✳
- Levaquin 750mg QD ✳
- Doxycycline 100mg Q12H (sinusitis) ✳
- Ceftin (cefuroxime) Q12H ✳

- Cipro 250-500 Q12H ✳
- Bactrim DS Q12H ✳
- Nitrofurontoin 50-100 Q6H

- Clindamycin 300mg Q6H ✳
- Keflex 500mg Q6H ✳
- Amoxicillin 500mg ✳
- Flagyl 500mg ✳
- Acyclovir 400-800mg

- Bentyl (Dycyclomine) 20mg Q6H ○
- Zofran (ondansetron) ODT 4mg Q8H ○
- Reglan 10mg ○

- Omeprazole ○
- Pantoprazole ○
- Ranitidine (Zantac) ○

- Ibuprofen 200-800mg Q8H PRN ○
- Diclofenac 50-75mg Q12H PRN ○
- Meloxican 7.5-15 ○
- Naproxen 250-500mg ○
- Colchicine 0.6mg max 1.8/day ○
- Tylenol 500-650mg Q6H ○

- Alendronate 70mg QWeekly ✳✳
- Caltrate TID ✳✳

- Tamsulosin 0.4 QD ○
- Oxybutinin 5mg BID ○

- Vit D 50000 units ✳
- Vit E 400units 2/Qam ✳

- Sertraline 25-200mg QHS ✳
- Duloxetine 30mg QHS ✳
- Fluoxetine ✳

- Topamax 25-200mg QHS ✳
- Maxalt 10mg Q2H PRN Max 30mg/day ✳

Labs

- Leukocytosis (High WBC)
  Recheck CBC (posible secondary to infection)
  - Hemoglobin low- Anemia
  Order anemia panel
    - Hemoglobin and hematocrit higher than 18 Polycythemia
  Order Chest X-ray PA and Lateral
  Possible secondary to lung condition, testosterone injection, smoking, OSA.
    - Thrombocytopenia (low platelets)
  Recheck CBC
  Send to Hem-onc if 2 times low
  If <50,000 send to ER
    - Thrombocytosis (High Platelets)
  Recheck CBC
  Send Hem-Onc
    - Elevated LFT's
  Recheck, Abdominal US, Hep Panel and AFP
    - Fatty liver
  Check yearly Abdominal US, Hep Panel and AFP
    - Cirrhosis
  Start 400units 2pills in AM

- Veltassa
  Lokelma
    - Hyperkalemia
    - Hypokalemia
  Give potassium PO
    - Alkaline phosphatase
  Fractionate ALK
  Recheck liver enzymes
  If bone elevation order a Bone Scan

  Liver Doppler
  Abdominal US

  Folic Acid 1g and Thiamine 100mg
    - Elevated Alkaline Phosphatase
  Fractionate it
    - Leukopenia (low WBC)
  HIV test and Hepatitis Panel

Preventive Medicine

- **Female and Male**
  STD panel (When sexually active) Yearly
  HIV >16y/o (even if not sexually active)

- **Female**
  Pap Smear 21> every 3years 21-29
  30-65 every 5years with HPV
  Mammogram 40> every year
  DEXA 45>
  Colonoscopy 45> every 10 years if normal
  FOBT yearly

- **Male**
  PSA 50> yearly
  DEXA 50>
  Colonoscopy 45> Q10 years if normal
  FOBT yearly

- ABI
- Arterial Doppler
- Venous Doppler
- EKG
- 2D Echo
- Pseudoscan
- Xray
- Abdominal US
- Pelvic US
- Transvaginal US
- CT
- Thyroid Us
- HIDA Scan
- Renal US
- Liver Doppler
- Spot compression
- Breast US

Add Diagnoses

Referrals & FU

- Podiatrist
- Ophtalmologist
- Cardiologist
- GI
- Pulmo
- Psych
- Counselor
- Neuro

- Orthopedic
- Pain Specialist
- Sleep Study
- Plastic surgery
- GI/Hernia
- repair surgeon
- Urologist
- Nephrologist
- OB/GYN

Follow up: _____

Labs

- Leukocytosis (High WBC)
  - Recheck CBC (posible secondary to infection)
- Hemoglobin low- Anemia
  - Order anemia panel
- Hemoglobin and hematocrit higher than 18 Polycythemia
  - Order Chest X-ray PA and Lateral
  - Possible secondary to lung condition, testosterone injection, smoking, OSA.
- Thrombocytopenia (low platelets)
  - Recheck CBC
  - Send to Hem-onc if 2 times low
  - If <50,000 send to ER
- Thrombocytosis (High Platelets)
  - Recheck CBC
  - Send Hem-Onc
- Veltassa
- Lokelma
- Hyperkalemia
- Hypokalemia
  - Give potassium PO
- Plumbism (lead poison >5mcg/dL)
  - Lead level (BLL) of 5 mcg/dL (Normal)
  - Chelation Theraphy
  - Refer to ER

Medications

Tylenol
Ibuprofen
Omnicef (cefdinir) 250mg/5ml
Augmentin 250/62.5mg
Doxycycline 25mg/5ml (sinusitis)
Ceftin (cefuroxime) 250mg/5ml

Cipro 250-500/5ml
Nitrofurontoin 25mg/5ml

Clindamycin 75mg/5ml
Keflex 125-250mg/5ml
Amoxicillin 125-400mg/5ml
Acyclovir 200mg/5ml

Bentyl (Dycyclomine) 10mg/5ml
Zofran (ondasentron) ODT 4mg/5ml

Ceterizine 5mg QD chew or 1mg/1ml
Montelukast 4-5mg QHS
Flonase 4-11yo 1puff QD >12yo 2puffs QD
Saline nasal spray PRN

Symbicort 1-2puff/BID
Albuterol Q4-6H PRN
Pro-Air Q4-6H PRN

Sertraline 25-200mg QHS/ Sol 20mg/ml
Duloxetine >7yo 20-60mg QHS only cap
Fluoxetine >6yo 10-60mg 20mg/5ml

Topamax >12yo 25-200mg QHS
Maxalt >6yo 5-10mg Q2H PRN
Max 30mg/day

Omeprazole
Pantoprazole
Ranitidine (Zantac)

Health Prevention/Orders

Female and Male
Lead Level (6,9,12,18,24 mo & 3-6yo)
CBC (if suspect anemia)
FBG & HA1C (>10)
Cholesterol panel 9-11/17-21
TB test (immigrants or exposure)
BMI % (>2)
Dietary/nutritional Counseling
Physical Activity
BP (>3)
STD panel (When sexually active) Yearly
HIV >16y/o (even if not sexually active)
EKG   Xray   Abdominal US   Pelvic US
CT   Thyroid Us   Renal US

Referrals

Ophtalmologist   Psych   Ortho
Cardiologist   Counselor   Nephro
GI   Neuro   OB/GYN
Pulmo   Sleep Center

_____

FOLLOW UP DATE

Vaccine	Birth	1 mo	2 mos	4 mos	6 mos	9 mos	12 mos	15 mos	18 mos	19-23 mos	2-3 yrs	4-6 yrs	7-10 yrs	11-12 yrs	13-15 yrs	16 yrs	17-18 yrs
Hepatitis B[1] (HepB)	1st dose	←——— 2nd dose ———→			←———————————— 3rd dose ————————————→												
Rotavirus[2] (RV) RV1 (2-dose series); RV5 (3-dose series)			1st dose	2nd dose	See footnote 2												
Diptheria, tetanus, & acellular pertussis[3] (DTaP: <7 yrs)			1st dose	2nd dose	3rd dose		←—— 4th dose ——→					5th dose					
Haemophilus influenzae type b[4] (Hib)			1st dose	2nd dose	See footnote 4		←— 3rd or 4th dose, See footnote 4 —→										
Pneumococcal conjugate[5] (PCV13)			1st dose	2nd dose	3rd dose		←—— 4th dose ——→										
Inactivated poliovirus[6] (IPV: <18 yrs)			1st dose	2nd dose	←———————————— 3rd dose ————————————→							4th dose					
Influenza[7] (IIV)						←———————————— Annual vaccination (IIV) 1 or 2 doses ————————————→								Annual vaccination (IIV) 1 dose only			
Measles, mumps, rubella[8] (MMR)					See footnote 8		←—— 1st dose ——→					2nd dose					
Varicella[9] (VAR)							←—— 1st dose ——→					2nd dose					
Hepatitis A[10] (HepA)						←——————— 2-dose series, See footnote 10 ———————→											
Meningococcal[11,12] (MenACWY-D ≥9 mos; MenACWY-CRM ≥2 mos)					←————————————————————— See footnote 11 —————————————————————→									1st dose			2nd dose

Printed in the United States
By Bookmasters